W0042763

Colorectal Cancer Screening

Han-Mo Chiu • Hsiu-Hsi Chen
Editors

Colorectal Cancer Screening

Theory and Practical Application

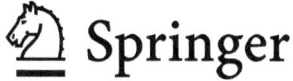 Springer

Editors
Han-Mo Chiu
Department of Internal Medicine
National Taiwan University Hospital
Taipei
Taiwan

Hsiu-Hsi Chen
Graduate Institute of Epidemiology
and Preventive Medicine
College of Public Health
National Taiwan University
Taipei
Taiwan

ISBN 978-981-15-7481-8   ISBN 978-981-15-7482-5   (eBook)
https://doi.org/10.1007/978-981-15-7482-5

© Springer Nature Singapore Pte Ltd. 2021
This work is subject to copyright. All rights are reserved by the Publisher, whether the whole or part of the material is concerned, specifically the rights of translation, reprinting, reuse of illustrations, recitation, broadcasting, reproduction on microfilms or in any other physical way, and transmission or information storage and retrieval, electronic adaptation, computer software, or by similar or dissimilar methodology now known or hereafter developed.
The use of general descriptive names, registered names, trademarks, service marks, etc. in this publication does not imply, even in the absence of a specific statement, that such names are exempt from the relevant protective laws and regulations and therefore free for general use.
The publisher, the authors and the editors are safe to assume that the advice and information in this book are believed to be true and accurate at the date of publication. Neither the publisher nor the authors or the editors give a warranty, expressed or implied, with respect to the material contained herein or for any errors or omissions that may have been made. The publisher remains neutral with regard to jurisdictional claims in published maps and institutional affiliations.

This Springer imprint is published by the registered company Springer Nature Singapore Pte Ltd. The registered company address is: 152 Beach Road, #21-01/04 Gateway East, Singapore 189721, Singapore

Foreword

Thirty-six years ago a valued mentor suggested that I assist him develop screening for colorectal cancer. He indicated that we needed a better understanding of occult bleeding from colorectal neoplasia and of the biochemical principles underlying effective detection using faecal occult blood tests. As a young gastroenterologist, this was not at first appealing to me because it was not an area that gastroenterologists, or surgical colleagues for that matter, were particularly interested in. I quickly realised that this was being shortsighted.

So, I took the advice of my mentor and embarked upon a long journey addressing research and clinical practice. During this time, there have been major advances in screening and diagnostic technologies as well as in the skill of the practitioners in diagnosis and treatment. Proof that we should go down this path came in the 1990s, when it was shown that faecal occult blood tests reduce population mortality from a disease which, by then, was affecting 1,000,000 people annually around the world.

It took a long time for practitioners, healthcare policymakers and providers to acknowledge the complexity of the multistep process required for a colorectal cancer screening programme to be successful in reducing mortality. Unlike some other screening programmes such as breast and prostate, the strongest advocates for colorectal cancer screening came from professionals, namely the gastroenterologists and surgeons, rather than from the public and support organisations. Public health experts gradually became more and more involved which meant that screening caught the attention of health policymakers and funders. And so, it became possible to move from the idea and evidence base to practical implementation within health services. In the last two decades, we have observed a global explosion from a basis where only a few countries were undertaking organised screening to a number in excess of 50 countries where screening has become public health policy and a national (or jurisdictional) priority.

Throughout this decades-long paradigm shift, the world has watched the colorectal cancer screening activities in Taiwan (the Taiwanese Colorectal Cancer Screening Program) with great interest. Taiwan was an early adopter of pilot programmes and the rolling-out of national programmes along with a few other countries such as my own. Early adopters like Taiwan stood out because internationally renowned public health experts joined with highly skilled practitioners and researchers to ensure that screening was done properly and feasibly within an existing healthcare structure. My own involvement with Taiwanese colleagues stretches back several decades as we have jointly participated in international networks and crucial publications that have helped advance screening around the world. Such work has gradually reshaped the initial, often naïve, plans as knowledge was gathered by careful observation of what was happening in practice. What has been impressive in Taiwan is that screening has been integrated across the professions and stakeholders from the outset of their pilot studies. Such are essential to test ideas that were largely theoretical at the start. They have their own population data, founded in a good information system, which has been drawn upon in this publication and which is hardly matched over such a long period by any other jurisdiction.

What the authors have set out to do in this book is to provide "a concise yet integrated instructional material" for those responsible for colorectal cancer screening. As they clearly describe in their chapters, this involves a very broad range of practitioners and a well-developed information system and data recording capability. They have effectively shared their experience to help guide others in establishing and improving their own programmes. Because this broad range of experts is well integrated in the Taiwanese setting, and because they have learned from each other, the guidance provided, both practical and theoretical, will be extremely useful.

The book delivers on the promise of its subtitle "theory and practical application". The justification for screening and the complexity of the colorectal cancer screening process are demonstrated by the topics covered in the 11 chapters. They describe how the multistep and multiskilled process is ideally coordinated within a public health environment, followed by practical issues around screening tests, their choice, and how they should be done. It also includes chapters on programme organisation and especially attention to quality. Experience shows that quality rather than quantity is the key to successful and ethically justified screening programmes. They also provide stimulating chapters on areas where their expertise in modelling and public health is particularly valuable, especially the basic theory on colorectal cancer screening with emphasis on natural history and the chapter on economic evaluation. But it must be noted that none of these theoretical issues are considered outside the practical considerations that are also necessary when embedding these in a public health organised programme within a country and when considering the other risk factors that apply. Importantly, they provide guidance on how one can start to go about personalising screening even in a national programme that seeks to optimally engage the relevant at-risk subpopulation. In the final chapter, they consider how screening might move forward in the future. It proposes models that are useful for this purpose, and it warrants careful consideration by all those involved in the implementation of such a health initiative.

This book is up to date and considers the challenges faced around the world. It demonstrates what one would expect from a country that is regularly ranked in the top ten healthcare systems and which has conducted an organised population-based screening programme for colorectal cancer for more than two decades.

This book is, therefore, going to be of relevance to those promoting health in the general field of cancer prevention and especially of colorectal cancer screening, to primary care practitioners who engage with people who should be involved, to those who assess personal risk, to all of the specialist practitioners particularly gastroenterologists, colonoscopists and colorectal surgeons, and to public health experts, screening programme coordinators and policymakers. It follows that if all of these groups work together in a cooperative and integrated fashion, screening programmes will be a success.

The authors are to be congratulated not just on their personal leadership in the Taiwan national programme, but also on having devoted the time and effort required to produce a most useful resource. This book demonstrates how much we have advanced in the last few decades in our understanding of how to get the best out of organised screening for colorectal cancer. It shows how a country with an excellent health service has done it, and it draws objectively on its own experience to guide the rest of us in what we could do next.

Graeme P. Young
Flinders Centre for Innovation in Cancer
Flinders University
Adelaide, Australia

Preface

Colorectal cancer has become one of the most emerging and threatening malignancies worldwide in the past few decades and more than 1.8 million incident cases are currently (2020) diagnosed every year according to the World Health Organization, and it has nowadays become one of the biggest clinical and public health challenges in developing and developed countries. In face of such a tidal wave of colorectal cancer, several effective measures should be taken. Among different approaches, screening has been demonstrated as one of the most effective ways to reduce mortality from this devastating disease and many regions have, therefore, launched population-based colorectal cancer screening programme in the past two decades.

Colorectal cancer screening, especially in the context of organised service programme, is pertaining to the coordination among different sectors of the healthcare community, including healthcare professionals, public health workers and health authorities of regional or central governments. As such, emphasising the importance of strategies that work through multiple settings and offering the opportunity of getting access to relevant domain knowledge gains increasing importance and is crucial for the success of a screening programme. Unfortunately, in the curriculum of medical school or continuing medical education in many countries, attention has been paid less to screening but much more to the diagnosis and treatment of colorectal cancer. Similarly, in school of public health, there are just a few courses dedicated to introducing screening theory and its applications. Meanwhile, we also felt the keen anticipation for such domain knowledge from our colleagues working in the frontline of the screening programme. We, therefore, came up with the idea of developing a concise yet integrated instructional material for our colleagues working in different sectors of colorectal cancer screening.

Our research team has been devoted to population colorectal cancer screening for more than two decades and in charge of Taiwanese Colorectal Cancer Screening Program since its pilot stage (1999–2003), launch of national programme (2004) and full rolling-out of programme (2010) till now. During this period, we worked in harmony with public health professionals, clinicians and government personnel and also accumulated tremendous amount of experience, information and know-how. Over the past few years, we have shared those harvests not only with the public heath students in the classes in College of Public Health of National Taiwan University but also with medical professionals and public health workers in serial workshops and the reaction from the audiences was very positive and sensational.

To be more organised and sharing those precious know-hows with more colorectal cancer screening personnel, we are determined to consolidate and rewrite the teaching materials and publish as a handbook.

We believe that the content of this book can fulfil readers of different healthcare sectors involving colorectal cancer screening. In Chap. 1, we briefly introduce the global epidemiological fact of colorectal cancer, and in Chap. 2, we address the differences of organised and opportunistic screening and analyse the advantages of the former from various aspects. In Chaps. 3, 4 and 5, we introduce colorectal cancer screening tests, including stool-based tests, endoscopy and novel blood-based tests. In those chapters, not only the screening tests but also their effectiveness on reducing CRC and its related death was introduced based on the currently available clinical evidence. In Chaps. 6, 7, and 9, we introduce the crucial issues in organised screening programme, including how quality assurance is conducted, what are the essential infrastructures for a screening programme, and how can the screening effectiveness be evaluated. This is of utmost importance for regions where screening programmes have already been in place but also provide useful information for those regions where population screening programmes are still in pilot or preparation stage, or about to start. Given that screening activities have been ongoing in many countries and people have now ready access to screening tests, it is still important to understand the ideas and rationales which lie behind them. In Chap. 8, we introduce the basic theory on colorectal cancer screening with special emphasis on its natural history and how it was applied in population screening. In Chap. 10, we introduce how the economic evaluation of colorectal cancer screening is performed. Owing to the funding and manpower constraint, such an issue is paid more and more attention especially in the context of population screening for selecting optimal and feasible screening strategy and allocation of limited resources. As lifestyle or various mankind risk factors are responsible for colorectal cancer risk to a different extent, screening should also be tailored stratified by different risk profile to maximise its effectiveness and minimise harm and make the most efficient use of the constrained resources. By applying big data and cutting-edge information technology, it is very likely that in the future colorectal cancer screening will take on a new look. In Chap. 11, we provide scope for the future of colorectal cancer screening from the viewpoint of big data and precision preventive medicine.

In the past 2 years, our authors have worked very hard to draft the materials in this book and tried to make the content both interesting and digestible. We expect that this book can fulfil the readers with different demands, including readers who are more interested in practical aspects and those who want to fill the gap between theory and practice as well as in relation to screening. We sincerely hope that our reader may feel the book useful and also feel our passion on colorectal cancer screening.

Taipei, Taiwan   Han-Mo Chiu
Taipei, Taiwan   Hsiu-Hsi Chen

Contents

Epidemiological Trends and Risk Factors of Colorectal Cancer: Implications for Population-Based Organized Service Screening

Sherry Yueh-Hsia Chiu and Chen-Yang Hsu

Abstract

Colorectal cancer (CRC) is one of the major global disease burdens that have been shown by the epidemiological time trends on both incidence and mortality rates. To ameliorate such a burden, early detection of CRC via population-based organized service screening program is effective in reducing colorectal mortality through evidence-based evaluation for population-based service organized service screening based on the indicator of mortality with a decomposition method.

Population-based organized service screening program is urgently needed in low- and middle-income Asian regions according to human development index (HDI) and CRC mortality in Western countries. To be efficient in the provision of population-based organized service screening programs in Asian countries with the rising trends on certain risk factors including smoking, less physical activity, and metabolic syndrome, personalized risk-based but still population-based organized service screening program should be considered given genetic susceptibility and family history. Such a personalized risk-based population-based organized service screening program is even likely facilitated by the expedient use of fecal hemoglobin (f-Hb) concentration that may have already capture individual risk profiles.

Keywords

Colorectal cancer incidence · Colorectal cancer mortality · Population-based screening program · Fecal hemoglobin concentration · Personalized risk-based screening

1.1 Introduction

1.1.1 Role of Population-Based Screening in Reducing Disease Burden of Colorectal Cancer

According to the GLOBOCAN 2018 estimates of colorectal cancer (CRC) incidence and mortality reported by the International Agency for Research on Cancer (IARC), there are over 1.8 million new cases and 881,000 deaths based on 20 countries'

S. Y.-H. Chiu
Department of Health Care Management, College of Management, Chang Gung University, Taoyuan, Taiwan
e-mail: sherrychiu@mail.cgu.edu.tw

C.-Y. Hsu (✉)
Graduate Institute of Epidemiology and Preventive Medicine, College of Public Health, National Taiwan University, Taipei, Taiwan

Master of Public Health Degree Program, National Taiwan University, Taipei, Taiwan

© Springer Nature Singapore Pte Ltd. 2021
H.-M. Chiu, H.-H. Chen (eds.), *Colorectal Cancer Screening*,
https://doi.org/10.1007/978-981-15-7482-5_1

information around the world. The incidence of CRC is ranked as third (10.9%) for males and second (9.5%) for females among common cancers. The corresponding rankings for CRC mortality are fourth (9.0%) for males and third (9.5%) for females.

There are three approaches (including primary, secondary, and tertiary prevention) to reducing mortality from CRC. Primary prevention such as lifestyle modification is to reduce the incidence of CRC through the elimination of risk factors responsible for occurrence of CRC. Secondary prevention (e.g., screening) is to reduce the incidence of CRC via the polypectomy of advanced adenoma through screening. The tertiary prevention is to improve case fatality through high quality medical treatment and health care. To reduce such a disease burden on the incidence of and mortality from CRC, one of the efficient approaches resorts to population-based organized service screening for colorectal cancer. A recent study (Lee et al. 2019), while decomposing mortality from CRC into incidence and case-fatality of CRC using Taiwanese cancer registry data over four decades by three age brackets, <50, 50–69, and 70+, found that the remarkable reduction of mortality was observed for the eligible screening population aged 50–69 years but not for the two other age groups without being invited to screen. These findings are entirely attributed to the magnitude of case-fatality reduction via, to a greater extent, early detection resulting from screening, and, to a lesser extent, tertiary prevention outweighs the increasing trend of incidence due to the lead time that advances the date of diagnosis for those in the absence of screening observed for those aged 50–69 years eligible for screening. Both the young age group and the old age group have seen the rising trends of incidence due to biological plausibility and aging, which outweigh the reduction in case-fatality due to the improvement of tertiary prevention through medical advances in treatment and therapy for CRC.

1.1.2 Decomposition of Epidemiologic Indicators for the Disease Burden of Colorectal Cancer

Mortality and incidence are the two indicators widely used as a fundamental tool for assessing the disease burden of colorectal cancer. Areas with elevated mortality and incidence are considered as the one suffering from the threat of colorectal cancer. The interpretation of these two indicators in assessing the status of colorectal cancer is, however, hampered by the counter-reciprocal effect of incidence and colorectal cancer survival. Furthermore, in countries with a mass screening program, these two figures can result in misleading information. With the rolling out of screening program, the colorectal cancer incidence is expected to increase due to the lead-time that advances the date of diagnosis of active identification of neoplastic lesions at their early stage by the program. These early colorectal cancers, compared with those being identified with clinical symptoms, carry a favorable prognosis and better survival, which will result in a decrease in colorectal cancer mortality following a sustained implementation of screening policy.

The provision of colorectal cancer screening programs is thus expected to bring down the mortality curve on population level. While evaluating time trends of incidence and mortality in relation to the benefit of screening, the targeted population should be limited to subjects eligible for attending colorectal cancer screening, namely, those aged between 50 and 69 years. Since the benefit of screening program can only be demonstrated among subject at this age band, these two common epidemiological indicators will perform differently across age bands in areas with a mass-screening program. Following this rationale, using crude mortality and incidence to assess the burden of colorectal cancer in areas with organized screening program thus results in misleading conclusions. The age-standardized rate, one of the most frequently used indexes in epidemiology, also leads to the erroneous results following the same rationale.

The time frame involved with the evolution of neoplastic lesions superimposed into the implementation of screening program render the use of mortality and incidence have further difficulty in assessing the disease burden of colorectal cancer. In the early years of screening program, the colorectal cancers identified in screening programs may close to the time of the development of clinical symptoms and thus have unfavorable survival. A transient surge in colorectal cancer mortality and incidence may be then observed in the early period of the implementation of mass screening programs.

Figure 1.1 shows the chronological trend of CRC mortality, incidence, and case-fatality for population aged 30 years or older. The three periods marked in the figure, (a) 1979–1994, (b) 1995–2003, and (c) 2004–2013, represents the epoch following the provision of National Health Insurance (NHI, since 1995) (Chan 2010), the inaugural period for the implementation of Taiwan Colorectal Cancer Screening Program (since 2004), and the rolling out period (since 2009) (Chiu et al. 2015a, Chou et al. 2015). The improvement in the accessibility following the provision of National Health Insurance with universal coverage resulted in the soaring in the mortality and incidence around 1995. Following the implementation of this national program in 2004, a transient increase in CRC incidence was observed, which was more prominent around 2009 with the rolling out of the program. In contrast to the soaring in CRC incidence, the mortality rate was stable after 1995. The consistent decrease in case-fatality was observed in Fig. 1.1c.

The chronological trend considering incidence, mortality rate, and case-fatality rate for the young (less than 50 years), middle (50–69 years) and old (elder than 70 years) age group are presented in Figs. 1.2, 1.3, and 1.4, respectively. Although the young age group had a lower disease burden, a similar increasing trend was

observed for the young as depicted in Fig. 1.2a, b. The chronological trend for the old age group was demonstrated in Fig. 1.4. The increasing trend in CRC incidence was similar but the mortality was plateau since the period after 1995.

Figure 1.3 shows the mortality, incidence, and case-fatality for the population aged between 50 and 69 years, which is the target population of Tawian CRC Screening Program. The increase in CRC during the years 2004 and 2009 was more prominent (Fig. 1.2b) as a result of mass screening programs. Notably, contrary to this soaring disease burden, there is a decreasing trend through the late period (2004–2012) compared with the middle period (1994–2013). The transient soaring in colorectal cancer incidence represents the process of active finding contributed from the national screening program. Although these CRCs were identified by the screening activity, they have been close to the time for the occurrence of clinical symptoms and thus the mortality in the corresponding period was fluctuating. Following these periods of lead time, a decreasing trend in mortality for this age group was observed with the sustained implementation of natioanl screening program.

From this illustration in Taiwan, the impact of mass screening program on the two major epidemiologic indicators, mortality, and incidence, can be demonstrated. The benefit of screening programs can only be evaluated by using a sufficiently long-term follow-up with adequate consideration of the time of program implementation and age groups eligible for attending the program. Through such an approach, the proportion of contribution to CRC mortality attributable to incidence and case-fatality can be quantified.

To address these issues, Lee et al. (2019) decomposed mortality into incidence and case-fatality by age groups with the consideration of population-wide interventions implemented in each epoch. The mortality was increased by 15% (95% CI: 10–21%) and 8% (95% CI: 6–11%) dur-

Fig. 1.1 CRC mortality (**a**), incidence (**b**), and case fatality (**c**) in population aged 30 years and older in Taiwan

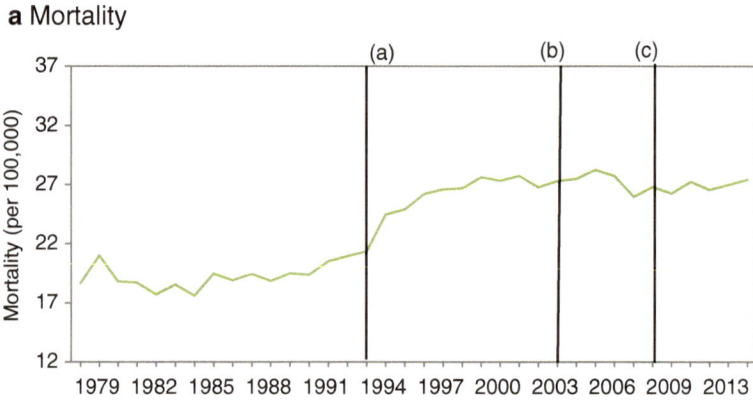

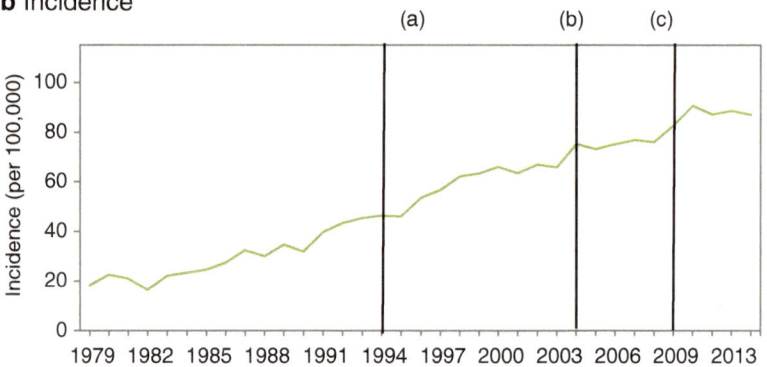

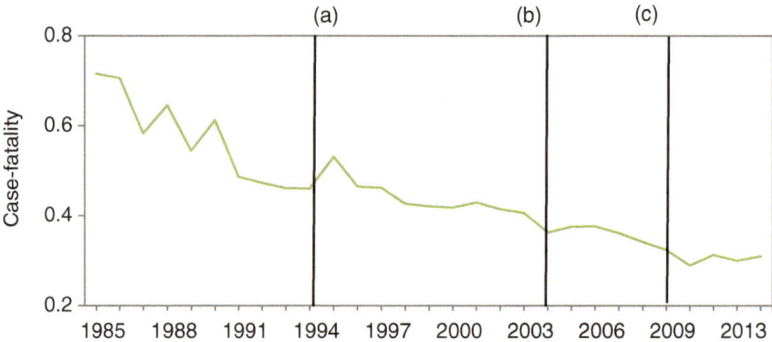

ing 2004–2013 for the young adult (less than 50 years) and the elder adult (older than 70 years) compared with 1994–2003. For the target population of the nationalscreening program (50–69 years), the reduction in mortality by 7% (95% CI: 5–9%) was estimated. Based on these results, Lee et al. further quantified the proportion of the impact associated with CRC mortality attributable to incidence and case-fatality rate. The result noted an increase in mortality attributable to incidence by 23% (95% CI: 21.7–24.2%) for the middle age group with the implementation of NCCSP. This effect was counteracted by the reduction in case-fatality by 28.3% (95% CI: 26.1–30.4%) due to early detection followed by effective treatment resulted from the national screening program.

Fig. 1.2 CRC mortality (**a**), incidence (**b**), and case fatality (**c**) in population aged less than 50 years in Taiwan

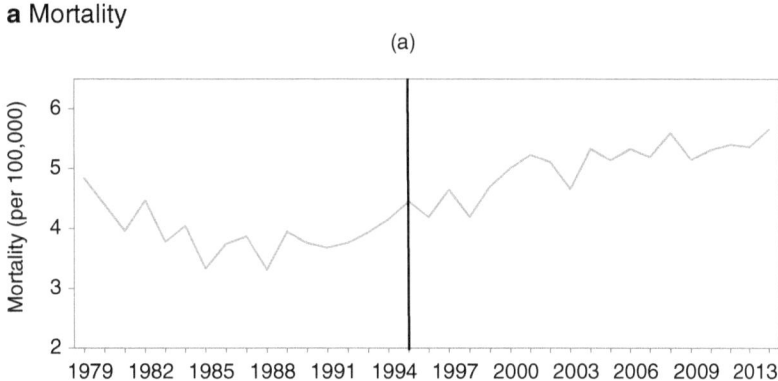

a Mortality

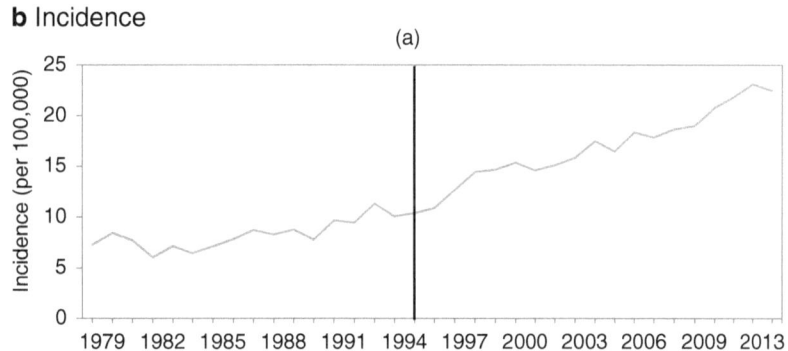

b Incidence

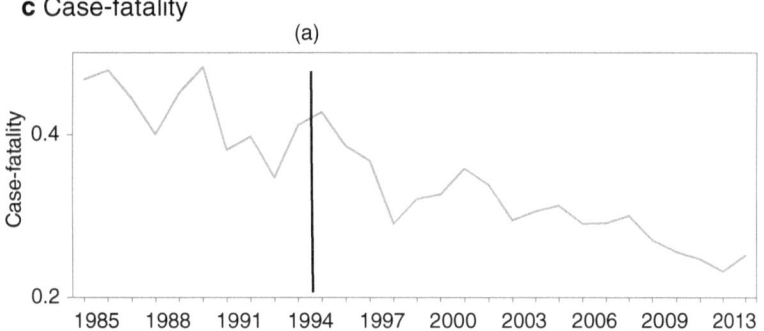

c Case-fatality

1.2   Socioeconomic Status and CRC

In addition to high disease burden at global level, there is a wide variation of age-standardized incidence rates (per 100,000) of CRC, ranging from the figure smaller than 5.2 to that larger than 22.8 based on data abstracted from the GLOBOCAN 2018. One of the key macro-level factors accounting for such a variation after adjustment for aging is pertaining to socioeconomic development. Generally speaking, the higher the socioeconomic status, the higher the age-standardized incidence rate (Bray et al. 2018). After analyzing the updated data from GLOBOCAN 2018, the positive association between CRC incidence and HDI was noted (Fig. 1.5).

Arnold et al. analyzed the long-term trend of incidence and mortality of CRC based on databases from Cancer Incidence in Five Continents

Fig. 1.3 CRC mortality (**a**), incidence (**b**), and case fatality (**c**) in population aged 50–69 years in Taiwan

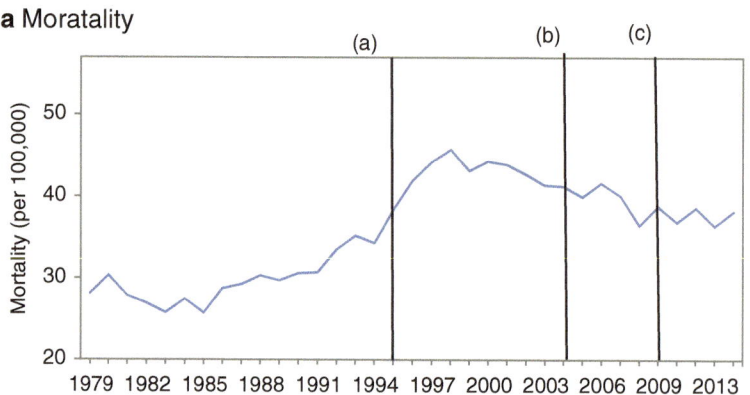

a Moratality

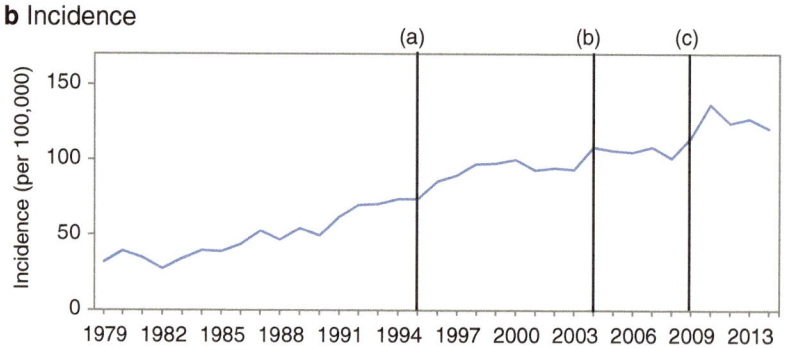

b Incidence

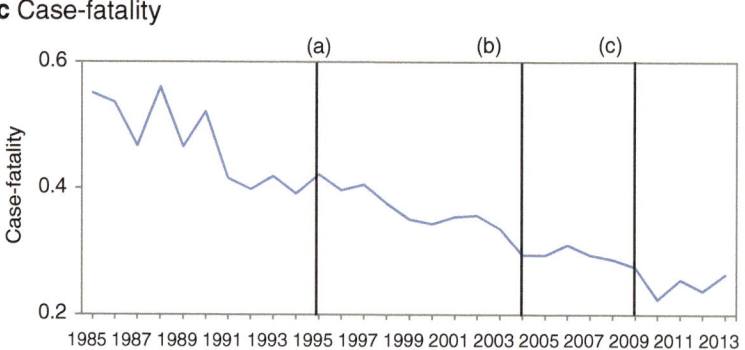

c Case-fatality

(CI5) to elucidate the temporal change in relation to the human development index (HDI). Three global patterns are classified by combining both CRC incidence and mortality of each country, including (1) the increasing trends for both incidence and mortality (e.g., China); (2) the increasing trend for incidence but the decreasing trend for mortality (e.g., UK); (3) the decreasing trends for both incidence and mortality (e.g., USA). For high HDI countries, the decreasing trend of mortality was attributed to good treatment and care and long-standing early detection screening program but the latter also contributed to the decreasing trend of incidence. As far as low- or middle-income countries are concerned, accessibility to treatment and care and screening seems very imperative to control the disease burden for the near future (Arnold et al. 2017).

Fig. 1.4 CRC mortality (**a**), incidence (**b**), and case fatality (**c**) in for population aged 70 years and older in Taiwan

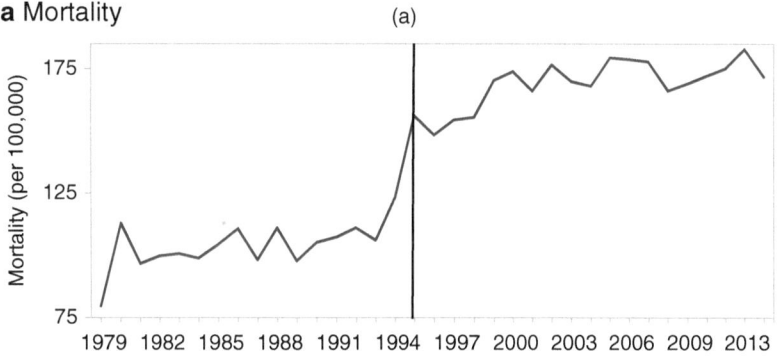

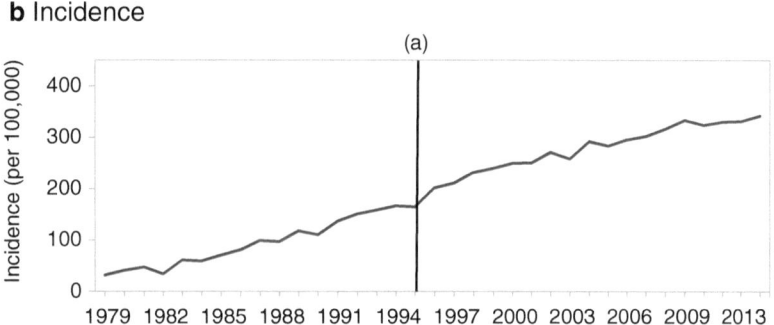

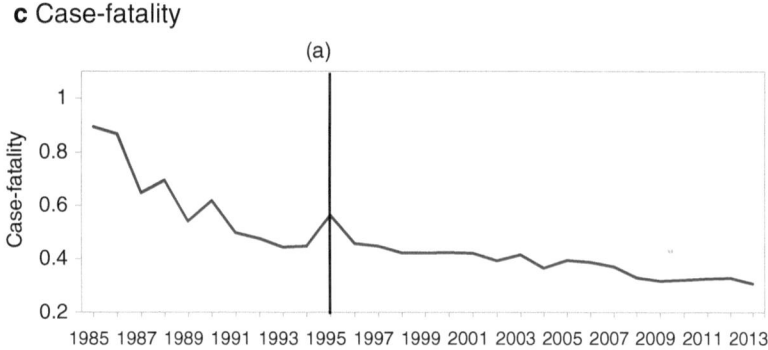

Besides three patterns, the increasing incidence of CRC in young adults was also noted worldwide. Based on US data analyzed by Siegel et al., the CRC incidence rate for those aged younger than 50 showed a double increase (2.4 times) based on the comparison between those who were born after 1990 and those born in 1950. Moreover, according to site-specific CRC incidence, one-third of those with rectal cancers were aged less than 55 years. Thanks to these findings, the guideline for CRC screening in the USA has been revised to recommend the starting age for screening commencing from 45 years of age (Siegel et al. 2017).

1.3 Colorectal Cancer in Asian Countries

The CRC incidence rates were even significantly divergent in Southeast Asian countries with the lowest and the highest incidence rates of 6.1 and

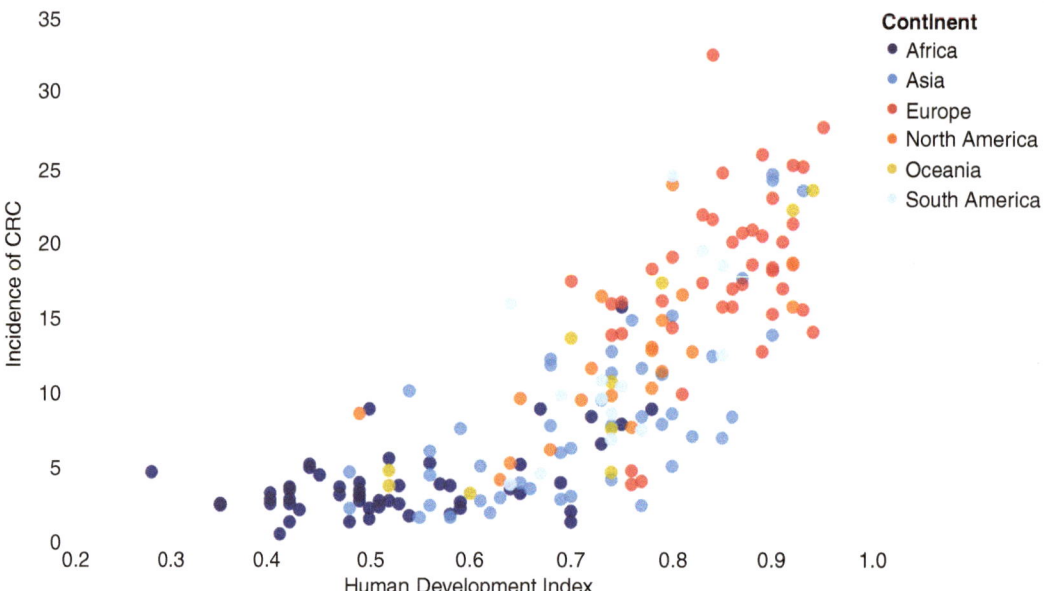

Fig. 1.5 The CRC incidence vs. Human Development Index in 2018

45.7 per 100,000 in India and Taiwan, respectively. For the economically developed countries in Asia, including Taiwan, Korea, Singapore, and Japan, the CRC incidence rates (45.7, 45.0, 33.7, and 32.2 per 100,000) were higher than others and close to those of the USA and UK. It should be noted that the CRC incidence rates in males were significantly higher than those in females regardless of the level of economic development of the countries.

According to the association between HDI and incidence and mortality and also our Taiwanese findings on the benefit of mortality focusing on those aged 50–60 years eligible screening as noted above, the implementation of population-based service screening would play an important role in reducing mortality and even incidence if early detection of CRC can be sustained for those low- and middle-income Asian countries.

1.4   Risk Factors for CRC

The risk factors responsible for CRC incidence include both environmental and genetic factors rather than one majorly dominated factor. The respective contributions to the occurrence of CRC were 60–65%, 23%, 5–10% of sporadic, family history, and hereditary cancer syndrome (e.g., HNPCC/FAP) (Reference, see Fig. 1.6), which revealed the majority of CRC sporadically arise from somatic genomic alternation. Besides the familial inherent genetic factors, so far, there is no conclusion on the specific carcinogenic exposure. According to some epidemiological studies, we give a brief on family history and some risk factors associated with CRC incidence.

1.5   Family History of Colorectal Cancer

Family history has been recognized as an important risk factor for CRC clinic, especially for the first-degree family relatives, which is important for identifying a high-risk population. The meta-analysis which combined 16 cohort studies demonstrated that a population with a family history of CRC was 1.80 times a significant risk of colorectal cancer incidence compared with no family history (Johnson et al. 2013) and the age of CRC onset for those with family history trait

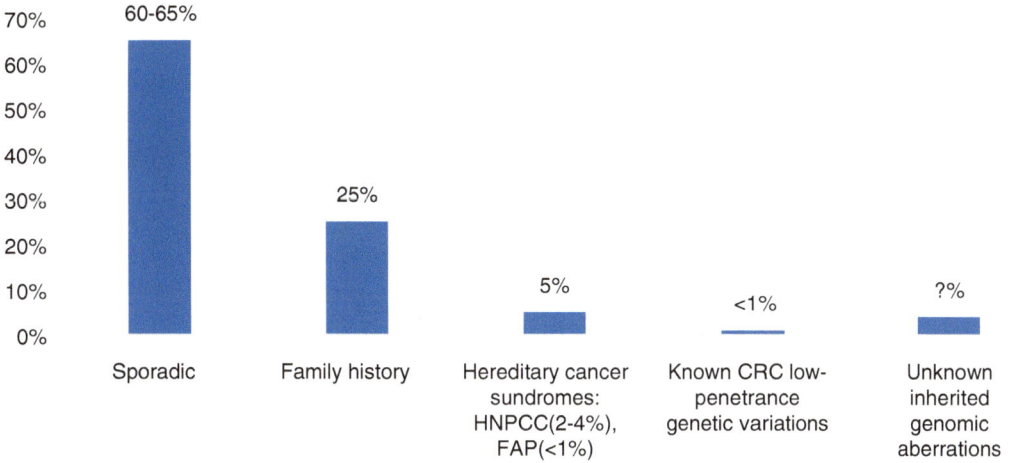

Fig. 1.6 Respective contributions to CRC associated with sporadic and hereditary factors (Redrawn from reference Keum et al. 2019)

was earlier than sporadic CRC. Specifically, on family history of colorectal cancers, it might indicate some diseases which are associated with family aggregation trend in CRC incidence, including familial adenomatous polyposis (FAP), Lynch syndrome (hereditary nonpolyposis colorectal cancer, HNPCC), MUTYH-associated polyposis (MAP), hereditary breast and ovarian cancer syndrome (Oh et al. 2018), and family history of sporadic CRC/adenomatous polyps. Both FAP and Lynch disease (Lynch et al. 1993) that belong to an autosomal-dominant syndrome are the highest risk for CRC incidence and strongly suggest that those need to have clinic surveillances with short interval using an advanced tool for follow-up. Even those high risks of CRC incidence, the knowledge, and awareness of the clinic surveillance might reduce the risk of being advanced CRC and having a better prognosis for CRC. In 2020, Pesola et al. conducted the Swedish National Colorectal Cancer Registry between 2007 and 2016 linked with multigeneration to identify the family or nonfamily CRC and to evaluate the survival rate. Those CRC young adult patients with family history demonstrated the early stage and better prognosis, which might be due to the high awareness of health and close/intensive clinic surveillance (Pesola et al. 2020).

According to the screening guidelines for CRC, the initial age for screening has been rec-

ommended at 50 years and 40 years for those with CRC family hsitory in their first-degree relatives; however, the natural history would be heterogeneous for different degree relatives. The risk stratification using polygenetic information is promising for early detection to provide customized screening and surveillance in the future (Henrikson et al. 2015).

1.6 Lifestyle and Exposures

1.6.1 Cigarette Smoking

Tobacco smoking poses a great threat to disease burden worldwide. The prevalent use of smoking has shifted from high- to low-income countries recently (Bilano et al. 2015). The meta-analysis in 2013 based on 12 epidemiological studies regarding the risk factors associated with CRC reported that high cigarette smoking was associated with a high risk of being CRC. Compared with nonsmokers, the relative risks were 1.06-fold (95% CI: 1.03, 1.08) and 1.26-fold (95% CI: 1.17, 1.36) for 5 and 30 pack-years, respectively (Johnson et al. 2013). Using the National Health Interview Survey (NHIS) with a cross-sectional household survey database consisting of 583,511 subjects from 1998 to 2017, Sanford et al. found, after adjustment for gender, ethnicity, and obesity, the adjusted odds ratio (aOR) for smoking versus non-smoking were 1.51 (95% CI: 1.10, 2.08) and 1.31 (95% CI: 1.20, 1.43) for subjects aged 18–49 years and >50 years, respectively. The higher impact was noted on the young adult (Sanford et al. 2020).

In addition to smoking on CRC incidence, Murphy et al., while organizing the European Prospective Investigation into Cancer and Nutrition study with 15 years follow-up, found the current smoking behavior had a higher risk of being CRC on the rectal and proximal colon in comparison with distal site (Murphy et al. 2019). Recent molecular epidemiological studies revealed that those who had MSI-high, CpG island methylator phenotype (CIMP) CIMP-high, and BRAF-mutant tended to have proximal CRC (Keum and Giovannucci 2019). The carcinogens from cigarette smoking have been conferred on cancer development through DNA mismatch repair (MMR) system, i.e., microsatellite instability (MSI) on risk of CRC incidence as those who had high MSI had significantly higher odds of being CRC by 1.94-fold (95% CI: 1.09, 3.46) compared with low MSI (Poynter et al. 2009). Carr et al. conducted a meta-analysis to elucidate smoking and MSI status associated with CRC. Based on three case-control and three cohort studies, those ever smokers had significant 1.62-fold (95% CI: 1.40, 1.88) risk associated with MSI-H CRC (Carr et al. 2018). As the prevalence of smoking has been increasing in middle- or low-developed countries, an increase in CRC incidence rate would be expected in the next decade. For early detection of the rising trend of CRC, risk-based population-based organized service screening for CRC would be highly recommended.

1.6.2 Obesity

Obesity has been established as a strong risk factor for CRC incidence that 11% CRC would be attributed to overweight and obesity (Bardou et al. 2013) that are related to the mechanisms through insulin resistance, chronic inflammation, or adipocytokines (Jochem and Leitzmann 2016).

Both measures waist circumference (WC) and body mass index (BMI) are applied for obesity criteria. Bardou et al. reported that an elevated 3% risk of CRC incidence was noted in parallel with 1 BMI increase and this effect was higher for men than women (Bardou et al. 2013). The dose-response effect of BMI on CRC incidence was also noted.

The CRC incidence rate of young adults has been steadily and continuously rising in this decade, but the etiological profiles are still poorly understood. Liu et al. used the long-term follow-up cohort, Nurses' Health Study II prospective cohort with 85,256 women aged 25–42 years, to investigate the obesity associated with CRC, The results showed the risks were 1.37-fold (95% CI, 0.81, 2.30) and 1.93-fold (95% CI, 1.15, 3.25) for overweight (BMI 25.0–29.9) and obese (BMI $\geq$ 30), compared with BMI 18.5–22.9 based on those young populations. The risk of CRC was increased by 20% per 5-unit increase in BMI (Liu et al. 2019). Sanford et al. reported a significant finding that BMI $\geq$ 30 led to an increase in CRC incidence by 1.39-fold (95% CI: 1.00, 1.92) for the young population, but not for those aged $\geq$50 years (OR = 0.93, 95% CI: 0.85, 1.03) after adjusting for other factors (Sanford et al. 2020). As the prevalence rate of obesity increasing in the world, especially on young adults, the primary prevention strategy for CRC should curb tide by weight reduction. Personalized risk-based population-based organized service screening targeting at subjects with obesity can be an alternative approach to reduce mortality from CRC in this group.

1.6.3 Physical Activity

Obesity is obviously an important risk factor for CRC incidence. On the other hand, some approaches to reducing fat or weight might show a protective effect on CRC risk. In 2016, Keum et al. found the Health Professionals Follow-up Study with 43,479 subjects to examine the relationship between physical activity and digestive cancer risk. Using the metabolic equivalent of task (MET) with hours/week, the significant inverse association was reported in a dose-response manner, high MET with low cancer risk (Keum et al. 2016). Shaw et al. conducted the systematic review with BMI and first-degree family history information to perform the meta-analysis on the association between physical activity and CRC risk. The effect of physical activity on reducing CRC risk was demonstrated with the significant effect noted for (OR = 0.56, 95% CI: 0.39, 0.80) first-degree family history, but not for those who were with (OR = 0.72, 95% CI: 0.39, 1.32) first-degree family history. In addition to family history, the physical activity also gave additional benefit of reducing risk among higher BMI (OR = 0.65, 95% CI: 0.53, 0.79) in comparison with low BMI (OR = 0.74, 95% CI: 0.66, 0.83) (Shaw et al. 2018).

The incidence rate of CRC has been steadily increasing in developed countries, especially for those aged over 50 years, which was covered by screening programs; however, the incidence trends for the younger population were significantly increasing with the evolution of birth cohort. The pattern in the early diagnosis of CRC tends to yield sporadic cases rather than those with family history. It is highly suspected that lifestyle changes and environmental exposures in generational change would play potential roles as risk factor (Stoffel and Murphy 2020). Lifestyles and exposures impact on CRC are varied for different countries due to the different frequencies and exposures (Onyoh et al. 2019). Therefore, the screening program may play a vital role in reducing both incidence and mortality rates of CRC for the young population. However, personalized risk-based population-based organized service screening may be needed as the absolute incidence for the young age is still low in comparison with the eligible screening population.

1.7 Metabolic Syndrome and Components Associated with CRC

Metabolic factors, such as obesity and diabetes, are well-known risk factors for CRC. The multiple-disease screening program was launched in Keelung, the northernmost harbor city of Taiwan, in 1999. In this program, not only colorectal cancer but also other chronic diseases such as diabetes or hypertension were screened concurrently. The results show metabolic syndrome (MetS) was significantly at greater risk for colorectal adenoma by 43% (RR = 1.43 (95% CI: 1.01, 2.02)) (Chen et al. 2004).

As multiple disease screening may find numerous asymptomatic cases, our evaluation system also included the estimation of comorbidity of diseases in each individual. Based on the results from integrated multiple disease screening program, the subjects with asymptomatic neoplasms were more likely to have comorbidity with at least one type of nonneoplastic chronic disease like obesity, diabetes, dyslipidemia, or hypertension compared with those without. The association between the occurrence of a neoplasm and the presence of comorbid nonneoplastic chronic disease was found to be statistically significant (OR = 1.64; 95% CI: 1.38–1.94 [P < 0.05]).

The major components of MetS include obesity, hyperglycemia, hypertriglyceridemia, low HDL, and elevated blood pressure, and traditionally it was linked to the risk of cardiovascular or cerebrovascular diseases. In 2006, Ahmed et al. used the Atherosclerosis Risk in Communities (ARIC) multicenter prospective cohort, which was established since 1987 and followed up till 2000 to revealed the impact of MetS on CRC incidence risk. The significant dose response was shown by baseline number counts of MetS components and the effect was stronger on men (RR = 1.78, 95% CI: 1.0, 3.6) compared with women (RR = 1.16, 95% CI: 0.6, 2.2). This finding provided the effect of MetS on CRC incidence based on the long-term follow-up (Ahmed et al. 2006). In Sweden, the Metabolic Syndrome and Cancer Project (Me-Can) with 578,700 subjects also discovered the effect of MetS on CRC with 12 years follow-up. A similar result with higher risk on men (RR = 1.25, 95% CI: 1.18, 1.32) compared with women (RR = 1.14, 95% CI: 1.06, 1.22) was also demonstrated (Stocks et al. 2011). In 2007, Chiu et al. conducted a study on the ethnhic Chinese population in Taiwan using both National Cholesterol Education Program

Adult Treatment Panel III and modified Asian criteria to define MetS and explored the association between MetS and colorectal neoplasm. For those who had MetS, the risk of colorectal neoplasm was 1.35 times (95% CI: 1.05, 1.73) compared with those without. The adjusted OR of MetS were 0.96 (95% CI: 0.67, 1.38), 1.62 (95% CI: 1.14, 2.30), 2.15 (95% CI: 1/40, 3.31) for distal lesion, proximal lesions, and synchronous lesions, respectively. Therefore, not only that MetS had a significant impact on the risk of colorectal neoplasm, it also impacted the clinical phenotype of those lesion with more proximally located and synchronous lesions (Chiu et al. 2007).The gastrointestinal diseases are common in the general population, but where the direction is, and the relationship between them is still not very clear. In 2012, Tseng et al. conducted a study that included 7770 participants from a hospital-based health checkup population to examine the relationships between diabetes and gastric, esophagitis, and colonic diseases. The significant high prevalence rate of diabetes was reported on gastrointestinal (GI) symptoms of colonic neoplasm (26.6%) compared with noncolonic neoplasm (16.5%). The diabetes status also affected the sensitivity of the fecal immunochemical test (FIT), with 70.7% vs. 81.7% for diabetes and non-diabetes, respectively. This study indicated that diabetes not only plays an important role in colonic neoplasm incidence but also influences the performance of a screening tool for CRC screening (Tseng et al. 2012). In 2012, the association between FPG or HbA1c and colorectal neoplasm were investigated base on the 2776 subjects with cross-sectional design. After adjustment for age, gender, and smoking, the adjusted OR was 1.22 (95% CI: 1.10, 1.36) for HbA1c, which indicates that the risk might increase 22% when one-unit increases of HbA1c. The HbA1c was significantly associated with colorectal neoplasm, but not seen with FPG. The meaning of HbA1c for long-term indicators revealed long-term control on glucose for diabetes cases is very important for medical care, which might reduce the risk of incidence of colorectal neoplasm (Hsu et al. 2012).

MetS is not only associated with the risk of colorectal neoplasm but also the risk of metachronous neoplasm after polypectomy. According to a study correlating MetS and metachronous or incident colorectal neoplasm, Chiu et al. demonstrated that compared with the non-metabolic syndrome (MetS), those subjects having MetS had a significantly increased risk of being colorectal neoplasms. The adjusted hazard ratio (aHR) were 2.07 (95% CI: 1.13, 3.81) and 2.34 (95% CI: 1.01, 5.41) for a normal and low-risk group (Chiu et al. 2015b).

Given that accumulation body of evidences demonstrating the association between Mets and colorectal neoplasm, we have to consider its potential impact and how it can be translated to CRC prevention. From the primary prevention perspectives, as MetS is a preclinical stage of chronic diseases, which are still reversible or slowing down of progression is still possible, intervention on those diseases may concurrently reduce the risk of colorectal neoplasms. From secondary prevention perspectives, the key components of MetS are also risk factors of colorectal adenoma, therefore, identifying individuals with MetS ties to the selection of individuals at risk of colorectal adenoma. For example, those factors of MetS can be applied to identify the high-risk population for a personalized screening program. The different intervals for different risk groups, namely the customized policy for disease management, would be made. In light of this approach, we successfully developed a novel integrated multiple screening model for the early detection of three nonneoplastic chronic diseases and five common neoplasms. Early findings from the Keelung Community Integrated Screening (KCIS) project suggest that outreach and community-based multiple screening programs not only enhanced the screening participation rate and also detected more asymptomatic cases for neoplasms and nonneoplasm diseases. From the viewpoint of research, this program provided a good chance of exploring the association between neoplasms and nonneoplastic diseases, furthermore, we could apply and translate those associations to high-risk identification efficiently.

Ku et al. assessed the causal relationship between metabolic syndrome on the risk of

CRC by using FIT as a surrogate outcome by using a population-based study (Ku et al. 2019). The study elucidated the temporal sequence of two strings of biomarkers, metabolic syndrome, and high fecal hemoglobin (f-Hb) concentration, both of which are related to the risk of CRC even after controlling for other confounding factors. Ku et al. used a bidirectional incident cohort study design to disentangle the bidirectional relationship between both and found MetS precedes elevated f-Hb (incident FIT-positive) but the opposite temporal sequence, i.e., elevated f-Hb leading to MetS is unlikely. Baseline MetS led to a statistically significant 31% (14%–51%) risk of being incident FIT positive. These findings suggest the control of MetS may contribute to reducing the risk of colorectal neoplasia. Given that f-Hbs have been demonstrated as the early biomarker for subsequent occurrence of CRC, our results suggest the control for MetS could be the core component for the primary prevention of CRC (Ku et al. 2019). The link between MetS and f-Hb from this study provides new insight into how to make use of f-Hb to design a personalized risk-based population-based organized service screening so as to capture risk profiles on main risk factors such as MetS.

In summary, this chapter begins with the epidemiological time trends on both incidence and mortality rates to reveal a global disease burden of CRC. How early detection of CRC via population-based organized service screening program is effective in reducing colorectal mortality is demonstrated through evidence-based evaluation for population-based service organized service screening based on the indicator of mortality with a decomposition method. Population-based organized service screening program is urgently needed in low- and middle-income Asian countries according to human development index (HDI) and colorectal cancer mortality. After a brief review of the risk factors in association with CRC, to be efficient in the provision of population-based organized service screening program in Asian countries with the rising trends on lifestyle factors and MetS, personalized risk-based but still population-based organized service screening program should be considered take into consideration the genetic susceptibility and family history. Such a personalized risk-based population-based organized service screening program is even likely facilitated by the expedient use of fecal hemoglobin (f-Hb) concentration that may have already been reported as a surrogate for individual risk profiles.

References

Ahmed RL, Schmitz KH, Anderson KE, Rosamond WD, Folsom AR. The metabolic syndrome and risk of incident colorectal cancer. Cancer. 2006;107(1):28–36.

Arnold M, Sierra MS, Laversanne M, Soerjomataram I, Jemal A, Bray F. Global patterns and trends in colorectal cancer incidence and mortality. Gut. 2017;66:683–91.

Bardou M, Barkun AN, Martel M. Obesity and colorectal cancer. Gut. 2013;62(6):933–47.

Bilano V, Gilmour S, Moffiet T, d'Espaignet ET, Stevens GA, Commar A, et al. Global trends and projections for tobacco use, 1990–2025: an analysis of smoking indicators from the WHO comprehensive information systems for tobacco control. Lancet. 2015;385(9972):966–76.

Bray F, Ferlay J, Soerjomataram I, Siegel RL, Torre LA, Jemal A. Global cancer statistics 2018: GLOBOCAN estimates of incidence and mortality worldwide for 36 cancers in 185 countries. CA Cancer J Clin. 2018;68(6):394–424.

Carr PR, Alwers E, Bienert S, Weberpals J, Kloor M, Brenner H, Hoffmeister M. Lifestyle factors and risk of sporadic colorectal cancer by microsatellite instability status: a systematic review and meta-analyses. Ann Oncol. 2018;29(4):825–34.

Chan WSH. Taiwan's healthcare report 2010. EPMA J. 2010;1(4):563–85.

Chen TH, Chiu YH, Luh DL, Yen MF, Wu HM, Chen LS, Tung TH, Huang CC, Chan CC, Shiu MN, Yeh YP, Liou HH, Liao CS, Lai HC, Chiang CP, Peng HL, Tseng CD, Yen MS, Hsu WC, Chen CH, Taiwan Community-Based Integrated Screening Group. Community-based multiple screening model: design, implementation, and analysis of 42,387 participants. Cancer. 2004;100(8):1734–43.

Chiu HM, Lin JT, Shun CT, Liang JT, Lee YC, Huang SP, Wu MS. Association of metabolic syndrome with proximal and synchronous colorectal neoplasm. Clin Gastroenterol Hepatol. 2007;5(2):221–9.

Chiu HM, Lee YC, Tu CH, Chang LC, Hsu WF, Chou CK, Tsai KF, Liang JT, Shun CT, Wu MS. Effects of metabolic syndrome and findings from baseline colonoscopies on occurrence of colorectal neoplasms. Clin Gastroenterol Hepatol. 2015a;13(6):1134–42.e8.

Chiu HM, Chen SLS, Yen AMF, et al. Effectiveness of fecal immunochemical testing in reducing colorectal cancer mortality from the one million Taiwanese screening program. Cancer. 2015b;121(18):3221–9.

Chou CK, Chen SLS, Yen AMF, et al. Outreach and inreach organized service screening programs for colorectal cancer. PLoS One. 2015;s11(5).

Henrikson NB, Webber EM, et al. Family history and the natural history of colorectal cancer: systematic review. Genet Med. 2015;17(9):702–12.

Hsu YC, Chiu HM, Liou JM, Chang CC, Lin JT, Liu HH, Wu MS. Glycated hemoglobin A1c is superior to fasting plasma glucose as an independent risk factor for colorectal neoplasia. Cancer Causes Control. 2012;23(2):321–8.

Jochem C, Leitzmann M. Obesity and colorectal cancer. Recent Results Cancer Res. 2016;208:17–41.

Johnson CM, Wei C, Ensor JE, Smolenski DJ, Amos CI, Levin B, Berry DA. Meta-analyses of colorectal cancer risk factors. Cancer Causes Control. 2013;24(6):1207–22.

Keum N, Giovannucci E. Global burden of colorectal cancer: emerging trends, risk factors and prevention strategies. Nat Rev Gastroenterol Hepatol. 2019;16(12):713–32.

Keum N, Bao Y, Smith-Warner SA, Orav J, Wu K, Fuchs CS, Giovannucci EL. Association of physical activity by type and intensity with digestive system cancer risk. JAMA Oncol. 2016;2(9):1146–53.

Ku MS, Fann JCY, Chiu SYH, Chen HH, Hsu CY. Elucidating bidirectional relationship between metabolic syndrome and elevated faecal haemoglobin concentration: a Taiwanese community-based cohort study. BMJ Open. 2019;9(3):e021153.

Lee YC, Hsu CY, Chen SLS, et al. Effects of screening and universal healthcare on long-term colorectal cancer mortality. Int J Epidemiol. 2019;48(2):538–48.

Liu PH, Wu K, Ng K, et al. Association of obesity with risk of early-onset colorectal cancer among women. JAMA Oncol. 2019;5(1):37–44.

Lynch HT, Smyrk TC, Watson P, Lanspa SJ, Lynch JF, Lynch PM, Cavalieri RJ, Boland CR. Genetics, natural history, tumor spectrum, and pathology of hereditary nonpolyposis colorectal cancer: an updated review. Gastroenterology. 1993;104(5):1535–49.

Murphy N, Ward HA, Jenab M, et al. Heterogeneity of colorectal cancer risk factors by anatomical subsite in 10 European countries: a multinational cohort study. Clin Gastroenterol Hepatol. 2019;17(7):1323–31.

Oh M, McBride A, Yun S, Bhattacharjee S, Slack M, Martin JR, Jeter J, Abraham I. BRCA1 and BRCA2 gene mutations and colorectal cancer risk: systematic review and meta-analysis. J Natl Cancer Inst. 2018;110(11):1178–89.

Onyoh EF, Hsu WF, Chang LC, Lee YC, Wu MS, Chiu HM. The rise of colorectal cancer in Asia: epidemiology, screening, and management. Curr Gastroenterol Rep. 2019;21(8):36.

Pesola F, Eloranta S, Martling A, Saraste D, Smedby KE. Family history of colorectal cancer and survival: a Swedish population-based study. J Intern Med. 2020;287:723. https://doi.org/10.1111/joim.13036.

Poynter JN, Haile RW, Siegmund KD, Campbell PT, Figueiredo JC, Limburg P, Young J, Le Marchand L, Potter JD, Cotterchio M, Casey G, Hopper JL, Jenkins MA, Thibodeau SN, Newcomb PA, Baron JA, Colon Cancer Family Registry. Associations between smoking, alcohol consumption, and colorectal cancer, overall and by tumor microsatellite instability status. Cancer Epidemiol Biomark Prev. 2009;18(10):2745–50.

Sanford NN, Giovannucci EL, Ahn C, Dee EC, Mahal BA. Obesity and younger versus older onset colorectal cancer in the United States, 1998-2017. J Gastrointest Oncol. 2020;11(1):121–6.

Shaw E, Farris MS, Stone CR, Derksen JWG, Johnson R, Hilsden RJ, Friedenreich CM, Brenner DR. Effects of physical activity on colorectal cancer risk among family history and body mass index subgroups: a systematic review and meta-analysis. BMC Cancer. 2018;18(1):71.

Siegel RL, Fedewa SA, Anderson WF, Miller KD, Ma J, Rosenberg PS, Jemal A. Colorectal cancer incidence patterns in the United States, 1974–2013. J Natl Cancer Inst. 2017;109(8).

Stocks T, Lukanova A, Bjørge T, et al. Metabolic syndrome cancer project me-can group. Metabolic factors and the risk of colorectal cancer in 580,000 men and women in the metabolic syndrome and cancer project (me-can). Cancer. 2011;117(11):2398–407.

Stoffel EM, Murphy CC. Epidemiology and mechanisms of the increasing incidence of colon and rectal cancers in young adults. Gastroenterology. 2020;158(2):341–53.

Tseng PH, Lee YC, Chiu HM, Chen CC, Liao WC, Tu CH, Yang WS, Wu MS. Association of diabetes and HbA1c levels with gastrointestinal manifestations. Diabetes Care. 2012;35(5):1053–60.

Population-Based Organized Service Screening for Colorectal Cancer

2

Szu-Min Peng and Sam Li-Sheng Chen

Abstract

This chapter first introduces the necessity of extending evidence-based colorectal cancer (CRC) screening illustrated with the stool-based screening methods into a service screening program. The concept and feature of opportunistic and organized service screening were then distinguished by the way of invitations to the targeted population eligible for screening, the infrastructure of information technology, timely follow-up, quality assurance, and the better tracking of clinical outcomes. We then provided a systematic review of the existing screening program with both structured opportunistic or population-based organized CRC screening across countries over the past 20 years. Detection modes of early and late detection of CRC as a result of the periodical population-based organized service screening are defined by attendance rate at each round of screen and cancer diagnosed between screen.

Key elements for the implementation of population-based organized service screening are summarized. These include high attendance rate via mobilization of community construction, the installment of an integrated information system, the construction of an accessible referral system, the enrollment of sufficient manpower for outreaching screening and clinical service, the provision of sustained financial support, the integration of national or regional health care policy, the guidance of evidence-based information, the integration of primary care system and medical insurance system, and the development of evidence-based evaluation.

To achieve the most cost-effective in CRC screening, we prefer the organized service screening to opportunistic screening in order to systematically conduct, monitor, and evaluate a series process of periodical screening program from invitation, the uptake of screen, referral, confirmatory diagnosis, surveillance, and treatment until to the follow-up of primary and secondary outcomes.

S.-M. Peng
Graduate Institute of Epidemiology and Preventive Medicine, College of Public Health, National Taiwan University, Taipei, Taiwan

S. L.-S. Chen (✉)
Research Center of Cancer Translational Medicine, Taipei Medical University, Taipei, Taiwan
e-mail: samchen@tmu.edu.tw

Keywords

Opportunistic screening · Organized screening
Colorectal cancer · Infrastructure

© Springer Nature Singapore Pte Ltd. 2021
H.-M. Chiu, H.-H. Chen (eds.), *Colorectal Cancer Screening*,
https://doi.org/10.1007/978-981-15-7482-5_2

2.1   Evidence-Based for Population-Based CRC Screening

Population-based screening for colorectal cancer (CRC) with emphasis on stool-based methods has increasingly gained attention since 1980. Three large-scale population-based randomized controlled trials were conducted to demonstrate the efficacy of reducing mortality from CRC in the USA and Europe. The Minnesota randomized trial on CRC screening with a guaiac-based fecal occult blood test (gFOBT) has demonstrated 33% and 18% mortality reduction for annual screening and biennial screening regime, respectively (Mandel et al. 1993). Two European randomized trials also reported a 15%–18% mortality reduction for colorectal cancer screening with gFOBT biennially (Hardcastle et al. 1996; Kronborg et al. 1996). Despite these three studies, whether the effectiveness of mass screening can be beneficial to reduce morbidity or mortality is highly dependent on screening uptake, diagnostic colonoscopy rate, the quality of screening tool, the selection of target population, preventive strategies, compliance with follow-up or treatment, and costs. These questions play important roles in the effectiveness of screening while the findings of evidence-based studies are extended to service screening programs.

2.2   Opportunistic Versus Organized Screening

The delivery of service screening for CRC may be achieved through opportunistic or organized screening pattern. The distinction between organized screening and opportunistic screening mainly relies on whether and how the eligible subjects are invited to screen, test-positive subjects are referred to have confirmatory process, and precancerous adenoma and early detected CRC can have subsequent periodical surveillance.

Figure 2.1 shows the flow of a CRC screening with fecal immunochemical test (FIT). The process includes three main steps: FIT screening, the referral of screening test-positive cases, and confirmatory diagnosis and the management of detected neoplasm. In an organized screening program, the initial step is to engage the target population for screening test. The second step is referral of screening test positive subjects for confirmatory or diagnostic exams. Surveillance for screen-detected neoplasms is then offered during follow-up and appropriate treatments and therapies would be provided for early detected invasive CRC. Each of the procedure must be met by a variety of providers. It also requires funding to implement CRC screening and the necessary infrastructure as key elements of screening (Rabeneck 2006). In opposite to the organized screening, opportunistic screening for the identification of CRC is a case-finding approach that depends on either the attitude and the value of general practitioner or provider on secondary prevention or patient awareness during their visits to health care institutes. In opportunistic screening, there are lacking invitation list, scheduled tests (periodic screen), organized referral to have a confirmatory diagnosis, well-managed surveillance, adequate treatment and therapy, and evidence-based evaluation.

The invitation lists in organized screening are spawned on the basis of population-based household registry, which includes the entire target population. If subjects are not included in the invitation list, individuals are still able to visit health care providers and seek for screening services through opportunistic screening. The major difference between the organized screening program and opportunistic screening with respect to evaluation is that the organizer in organized program is able to measure coverage rate, referral rate, key quality indicators, compliance with surveillance examination, and, most importantly, the evaluation of screening effectiveness. As mentioned above, these characteristics may affect the effectiveness of screening, each step within screening flow should be managed and monitored. The benefits of screening would not be achieved if the quality on any step of the screening process cannot be ensured. From this perspective, organized screening, as opposed to opportunistic screening, enables one to have

Fig. 2.1 The flow of a FIT-based organized CRC screening

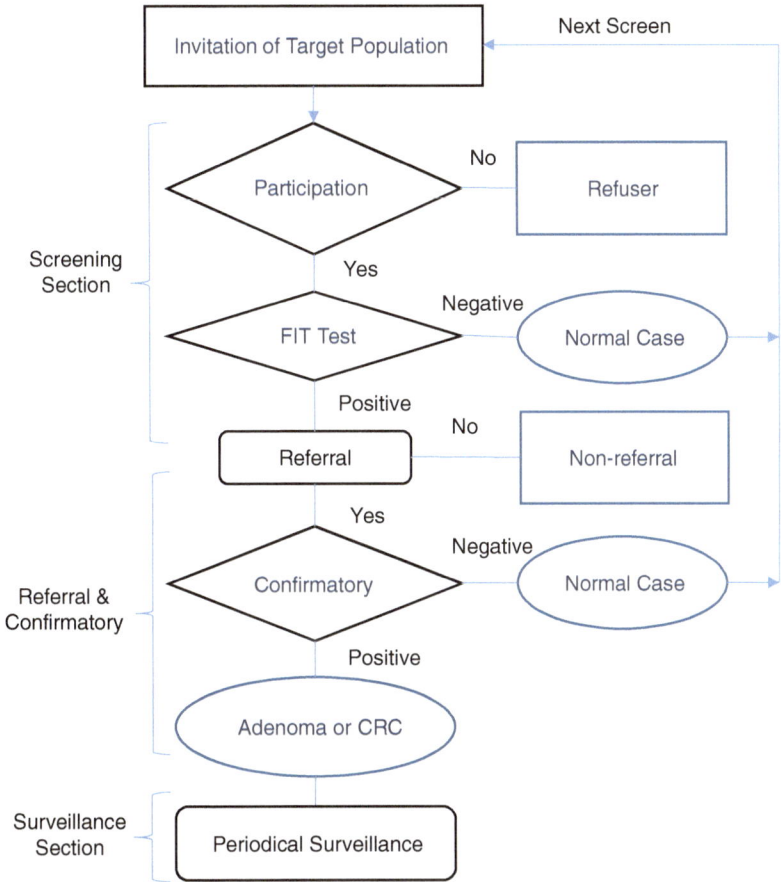

better-controlled procedures so as to maximize the efficiency, effectiveness, and even cost-effectiveness of screening.

2.3 Existing Screening Programs Worldwide

Table 2.1 summarizes the current types of CRC screening by countries. Except for Malaysia and the Philippines, most of the programs in the Asia Pacific belong to the style of organized screening whereas the screening programs in the United States, Poland, and Germany are based on opportunistic screening. Generally speaking, opportunistic screening is not centrally coordinated by a dedicated screening organizer and multiple options for screening tests can be recommended by the physicians or individual's willingness. Moreover, although call–recall systems or the

mechanism of quality assurance may exist in those opportunistic programs, the screening indicators (i.e., the uptake of screening, compliance with colonoscopy, or colonoscopy quality indicators) may not be regularly monitored and audited therefore the overall quality of screening might vary from country to country. Moreover, in opportunistic screening, benefit or effectiveness is more difficult to evaluate because different screening tests with irregular screening interval are used, and individuals can also change from one screening test to the other, and there is lacking central screening database integrated with other databases pertaining to the primary outcomes (cancer or death registry). The major advantage of opportunistic screening is that individuals have higher level of autonomy and more options for screening tests, but this may sometimes compromise the effectiveness and perhaps cost-effectiveness of the administration of screen-

Table 2.1 Organized or opportunistic screening for CRC by country

Country	Screening program type	Program	Age range (year)	References
Korea	Organized full	FIT	≥50	Choi et al. (2012), Schreuders et al. (2015)
Japan	Organized full	FIT	≥40	Schreuders et al. (2015), Sano et al. (2016), Ministry of Health, Labour and Welfare, Japan (n.d.)
China	Organized (regional)	FIT	40–74	Schreuders et al. (2015), Cai et al. (2009, 2019)
Hong Kong	Organized full	FIT	50–75	Schreuders et al. (2015), Cai et al. (2019), Benson et al. (2008), Chiu et al. (2017), Onyoh et al. (2019), Department of Health – Prevent Colorectal Cancer (Hong Kong) (n.d.)
Taiwan	Organized full	FIT	50–74	Schreuders et al. (2015), Chiu et al. (2015), Health Promotion Administration, Ministry of Health and Welfare, Taiwan (n.d.)
Australia	Organized full	FIT	50–74	Forbes et al. (2006), Cole et al. (2007), Senore et al. (2015), Australian National Bowel Cancer Screening Program (n.d.)
USA	Opportunistic	Colonoscopy, FIT	50–74	Senore et al. (2015), Division of Cancer Prevention and Control, Centers for Disease Control and Prevention, United States (n.d.)
Canada	Organized full (Province-wide)	gFOBT/FIT	50–74	Schreuders et al. (2015), Senore et al. (2015), Tinmouth et al. (2015), Canadian Cancer Society – Screening for Colorectal Cancer (n.d.)
Belgium	Organized full	FIT	50–74	Van Roosbroeck et al. (2012), Belgium Colon Cancer screening (n.d.), Association of European Cancer Leagues – Cancer Prevention (n.d.), Bowel cancer screening, International Agency for Research on Cancer, WHO (n.d.)
Italy	Organized full	FIT/FS	50–70/58–69	Association of European Cancer Leagues – Cancer Prevention (n.d.), Bowel cancer screening, International Agency for Research on Cancer, WHO (n.d.), Giorgi Rossi et al. (2011), European Colorectal Cancer Screening Guidelines Working Group et al. (2013), The Reference Centre for Epidemiology and Cancer Prevention in Piemonte, Italy (n.d.)
Spain	Organized full	FIT	50–74	Australian National Bowel Cancer Screening Program (n.d.), Division of Cancer Prevention and Control, Centers for Disease Control and Prevention, United States (n.d.), Tinmouth et al. (2015), Canadian Cancer Society – Screening for Colorectal Cancer (n.d.), Van Roosbroeck et al. (2012), Belgium Colon Cancer screening (n.d.), Association of European Cancer Leagues – Cancer Prevention (n.d.), Bowel cancer screening, International Agency for Research on Cancer, WHO (n.d.), Giorgi Rossi et al. (2011), European Colorectal Cancer Screening Guidelines Working Group et al. (2013), The Reference Centre for Epidemiology and Cancer Prevention in Piemonte, Italy (n.d.), Courtier et al. (2002)
Israel	Organized full	gFOBT/FIT	50–74	Schreuders et al. (2015), Senore et al. (2015), Levi et al. (2011), Abu-Freha (2019)
Netherlands	Organized full	FIT	55–75	Association of European Cancer Leagues – Cancer Prevention (n.d.), Bowel cancer screening, International Agency for Research on Cancer, WHO (n.d.), Navarro et al. (2017), Colorectal cancer screening programme (n.d.)

Table 2.1 (continued)

Country	Screening program type	Program	Age range (year)	References
UK	Organized full	gFOBT/FIT	50–75	Senore et al. (2015), Libby et al. (2011), Digby et al. (2013), NHS bowel cancer screening (BCSP) programme (n.d.)
Scotland	Organized full	FOBT/FIT	50–74	Swan et al. (2012), Bowel Screening (n.d.), Scottish Bowel Screening Programme, Public Health Scotland (n.d.)
Poland	Opportunistic	Colonoscopy	55–64	Senore et al. (2015), Boguradzka et al. (2014), Kaminski et al. (2015), Bugajski et al. (2019)
Croatia	Organized full	gFOBT	50–74	Abu-Freha (2019), NHS bowel cancer screening (BCSP) programme (n.d.), Bugajski et al. (2019), Katičić et al. (2012), Strnad and Šogorić (2014)
France	Organized full	gFOBT	45–74/50–74	Benson et al. (2008), Association of European Cancer Leagues – Cancer Prevention (n.d.), Bowel cancer screening, International Agency for Research on Cancer, WHO (n.d.), Navarro et al. (2017), Santé Publique France – National colo rectal cancer screening programme (n.d.)
Czech Republic	Organized full	gFOBT/FIT	≥50	Association of European Cancer Leagues – Cancer Prevention (n.d.), Bowel cancer screening, International Agency for Research on Cancer, WHO (n.d.), Navarro et al. (2017), Suchanek et al. (2014)
Germany	Opportunistic	gFOBT/ colonoscopy	≥50	Schreuders et al. (2015), Swan et al. (2012)
Latvia	Opportunistic	FOBT/FIT	≥50	Schreuders et al. (2015), Swan et al. (2012)
Lithuania	Organized full	FIT	50–74	Navarro et al. (2017), Poskus et al. (2015)

ing (Table 2.2). Only with organized way of screening then we can deliver high-quality mass screening to the entire eligible population given constrained manpower and funding resource (Dubé 2018; Rabeneck et al. 2020).

2.4 Periodical Population-Based Organized Service Screening for CRC

Population-based organized service screening is periodical and have a regular inter-screening interval. As it is affected by attendance rate at each round of screen, four types of detection modes are defined under the context periodical population-based organized service screening program, including prevalent screen-detected CRCs, subsequent screen-detected CRCs, interval CRCs (CRCs occur in between screening

rounds), and CRCs from refusers (CRCs occur in those who decline screen). As per definition, prevalent and subsequent screen-detected CRCs were asymptomatic CRC and detected by screening activity. Interval CRCs and CRCs in refusers are symptomatic CRC (Fig. 2.2).

1. Prevalent screen-detected CRC

    Based on information derived from the invitation list and history of screening, those who had positive findings from stool-based tests and diagnosed as CRC during the first screening round are defined as prevalent screen-detected CRC, which can usually be verified by linking screening database to cancer registry database.

2. Subsequent screen-detected CRC

    For the screening scenario in implementation, repeated screening should be engaged in a fixed screening interval based on the policy

Table 2.2 Comparisons of organized and opportunistic screening

Structure/process/ outcome	Opportunistic screening	Organized screening
Structure		
Setting and approach	• Clinics or hospitals • Case-finding	• Certified screening units or centers • Outreach screening service
Manpower	• None-specific or extra manpower	• Speficic health care workers • Well-trained manpower
Health care system on insurance and payment	• Paid by the health insurance company or pocket money	• Most financial support from the government • Cover low social economic area • Information technology infrastructure
Process		
Invitation	• No invitation or invitation by chance	• Targeted at eligible population • Standard and organized invitations by mail or telephone • Recall system
Referral	• Upon general practice	• Follow-up test • Timely arrangement • Quality assurance program (Credentialing of endoscopist, measurement of colonoscopy, adverse events, measurement of proportion of incomplete colonoscopies)
Surveillance	• Unscheduled surveillance • Awareness from patients	• Scheduled surveillance • Timely recall system
Treatment protocol	Following treatment guideline	Following treatment guideline
Outcome		
Program sensitivity	• Not available	• Available for assessment
Advanced CRC	• Hard to assess	• Available for assessment
Mortality	• Hard to assess	• Available for assessment

of a program. Compared with prevalent screening-detected CRC, those who had previous screening history with negative test, those CRCs detected at subsequent screening rounds are defined as subsequent screen-detected CRC, which can also be identified by linking screening database to cancer registry databases.

3. Interval CRC

   Those subjects with negative findings from the stool tests in previous screening but diagnosed as CRC with clinical symptoms before the next screening round are defined as interval cancers (in FIT screening program it is called *FIT interval cancer*), which might arise from missed CRC due to insufficient performance of screening tool or newly developed CRCs. For those who received colonoscopy and developed CRCs thereafter but before the recommended surveillance interval (usually rec-

ommended surveillance intervals are 10 years for a negative colonoscopy, 5 years for low-risk adenoma, and 3-years for high-risk adenoma), it is called *colonoscopy interval cancers* (Sanduleanu et al. 2015). Interval cancer is an important surrogate indicator for the performance of screening, especially when incidence or mortality data are still not available. The more interval cancers, the lower the program sensitivity is. In this view, cancer registry plays an important role in the provision of information on interval cancer arising from a periodical screening program.

4. CRC from refusers

   For those who are eligible for screening but declined any screening test and diagnosed as symptomatic CRCs later are defined as CRCs from refusers. It can be also identified by linking screening databases to cancer registry database.

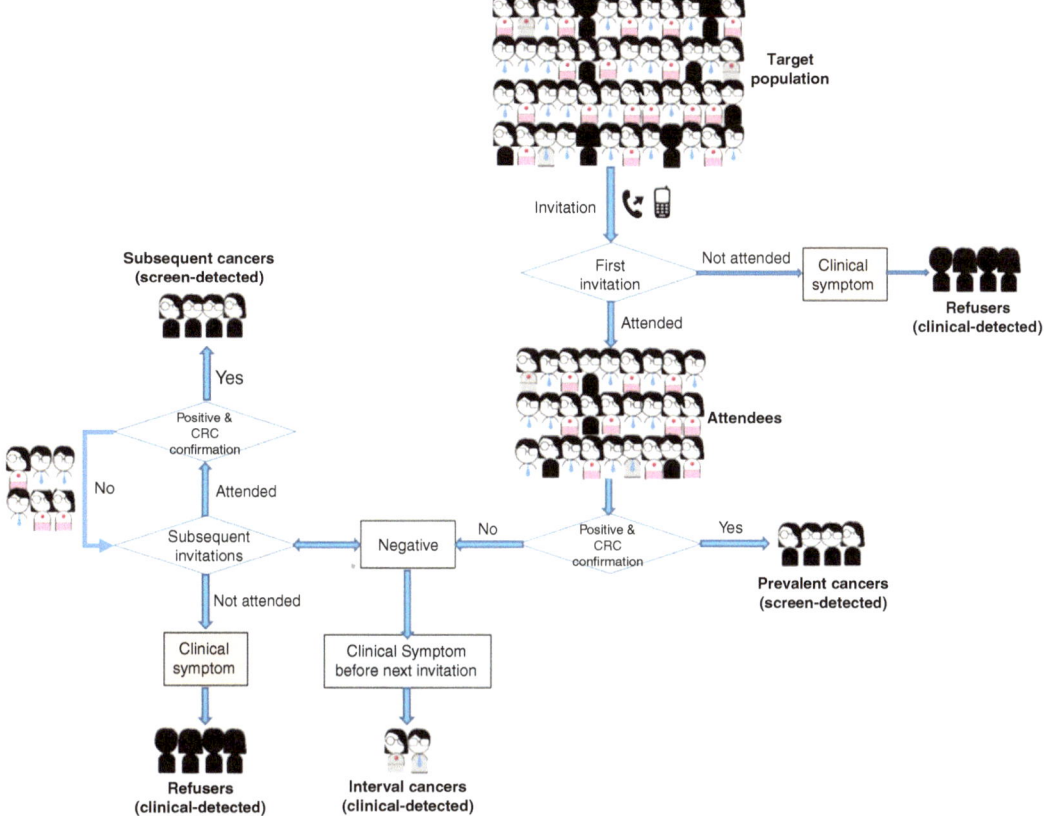

Fig. 2.2   The screening processes and detection modes in population-based organized service screening

2.5   Basic Elements in a Population-Based CRC Organized Service Screening

Implementation of periodical population-based organized service screening is a complicated task because it requires the formulation of an ecosystem rather than just implementing a single program or project. In other words, the purpose of implementing a population-based organized screening is to build up an interface that articulates various key elements pertaining to screening service. These include high attendance rate via mobilization of community construction, the construction of a comprehensive and integrated information system, the construction of an accessible referral system, the enrollment of sufficient manpower for outreaching screening and clinical service, the provision of sustained financial support, the integration of national or regional health care policy, the guidance of evidence-based information, and the integration of primary care system and medical insurance system. The key elements of population-based CRC screening are diagrammed in Fig. 2.3.

2.5.1   National Health Policy

In order to consider the feasibility of carrying out certain population CRC screening strategy, the organizers of screening have to firstly select the optimal screening methods based on screening theory, existent evidences and available resources, and then integrate with the current national prevention policy, such as existing organized or opportunistic health checkups offered by the regional or central governments by means of

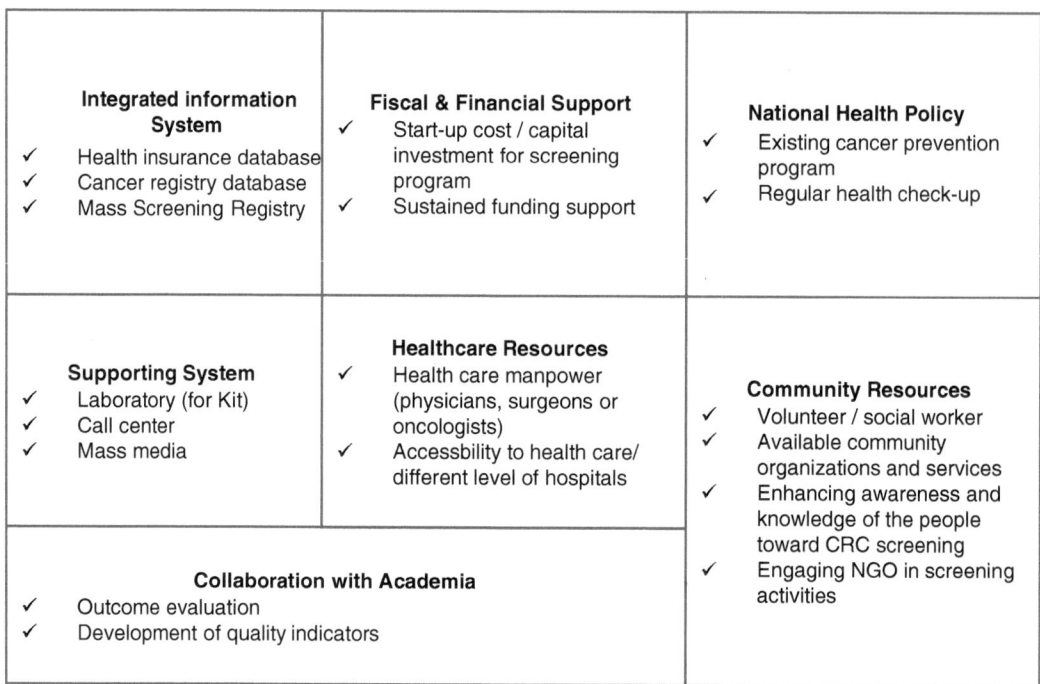

Fig. 2.3 The infrastructure with basic elements for a CRC screening program

liaison with different governmental departments and/or legislation. In addition, obligating hospitals to report ascertained cancers to cancer registry, which is indispensable for accurate evaluation of the screening effectiveness, also requires legislation. Take Taiwan for example, *Cancer Control Act* was enacted in 2003, 1 year prior to the launch of the national CRC screening program thereby provide the legal basis to integrate resources required for screening, obligate reporting of screening related information by individual health care institutes, and evaluation of the screening program in terms of quality and effectiveness (Cancer Control Act 2003). Formulating screening guidelines is another useful approach to leverage people to go for screening and provide a practical guide for physicians to follow.

2.5.2 Financial Support

Funding support is crucial for the sustainable development of a population-based screening program therefore screening organizers should strive for securing perpetual financial source. The screening program must also consider the exist-

ing prevention program and try to direct or integrate it into the newly developing one to avoid crowding-out of resources or the redundancy of similar activities. Undoubtfully this could be a thorny issue for the implementation of new screening programs because financial resources of new programs may come from central government, whereas other existent screening programs may be funded by the regional government, research projects, or other nongovernment organizations (NGOs). Practically, the financial support can start from a small research project for a pilot screening, and then upgrade to large-scale funding earmarked for a national program.

2.5.3 Health Care Resources

Taking the inventory of medical resources and reallocation of them before launching a population of CRC screening is crucial. Pre-planning of predictable manpower demand along with rolling out or popularity of screening with resultant increase in laboratory workload, colonoscopy demand, and clinical capacity to manage screen-detected neoplasms is mandatory for the smooth

Fig. 2.4 Different manpower required for CRC screening

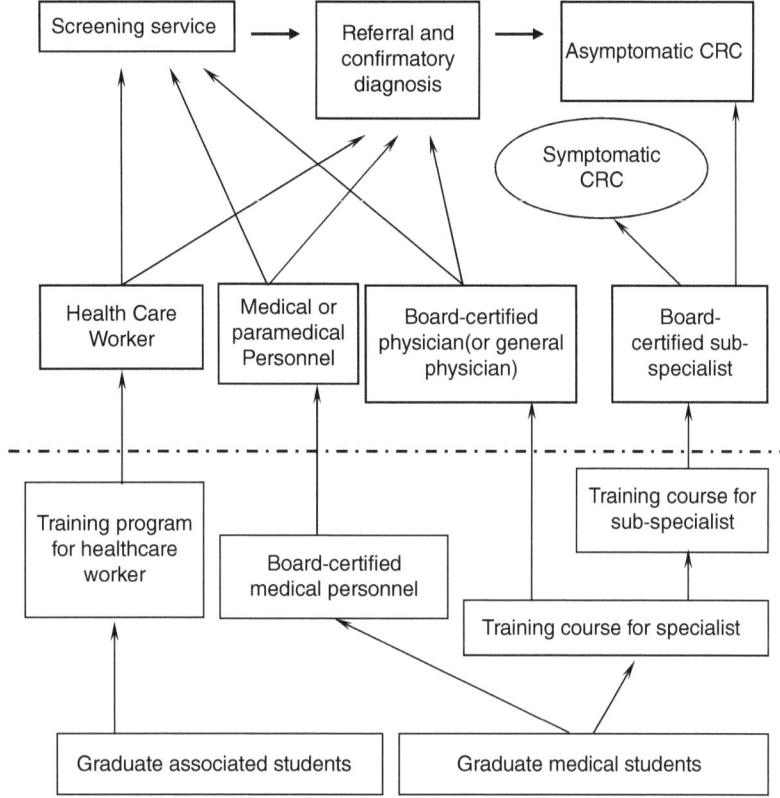

implementation of a CRC screening program. In the Taiwanese program, we have encountered a drastic increase in demand for colonoscopy when the program was extensively rolled out in 2009, 5 years after its launch, with resultant tripled number of positive FIT and increased demand for colonoscopy, prolonged queue for colonoscopy, and subsequently decreased colonoscopy rate (Chou et al. 2016; Jen et al. 2019). It was 3 years later that the colonoscopy rate recovered gradually from 50% to 70% after adjustment of screening logistics and liaison with professional societies and hospital authorities. Demand for professional manpower, such as gastroenterologist, surgeon, or oncologists, for screening procedures and the further management of screening detected neoplasm can also be provided on the basis of the parameters obtained from the results of pilot study results, current manpower capacity and the local trend of CRC epidemiology. Projection from such simulation may help cultivation and deployment of necessary manpower by the screening organizers and professional

societies (Seeff et al. 2004; Nnoaham and Lines 2008; Joseph et al. 2016).

Corresponding to the demand model for screening, CRC screening service in the workforce, the supply is provided by health care workers, medical personnel, and different types of board-certified physicians or general physicians (Fig. 2.4).[1]

---

[1]Medical personnel, including nursing staffs, medical technicians, and pharmacists, are determined by the supply of various board-certified medical staff, which are, in turn, affected by the supply of corresponding graduate students. The supply of board-certified physicians is pivotal in how they are supplied from internists or general surgeons, which also originates from the flow of general physician training after graduation from medical school, and gastroenterology or surgery sub-specialty training. If the targeted population is screened with FIT, those who receive FIT tests are defined as screenees, and those who do not receive FIT are classified as screen refusers. If a screenee has a positive result of FIT, then he or she will be referred for diagnostic colonoscopy to confirm whether further management is needed. After histological or radiological confirmation, further treatment, either polypectomy or surgery, or even systemic therapy would be provided.

2.5.4 Community Resources

In order to empower people to be endowed with the recognition that everyone has the responsibility and obligation to stay healthy, screening programs should not only provide services for people but also enhance the awareness of the people toward CRC and encourage people to take part in the health promotion activity such as screening. These include the persuasion of the key opinion leaders in the community to participate in screening activity, the recall of volunteer community social workers to get involved in screening activities, and the engagement of nongovernmental organizations (NGOs) to participate in the screening enlightenment activities or propaganda.

2.5.5 Supporting System Outside Ordinary Health Care System

Supporting systems other than ordinary health care system plays a pivotal role in screening, especially when screening takes place in outreach setting. In contrast to other cancer screening programs, CRC screening is rather complicated, as it has multiple steps, including engaging people to go for FIT screening, referral of FIT positive subjects to receive diagnostic examination like colonoscopy, which is invasive and requires complicated bowel preparation process, and conscious sedation during the procedure, and advocation of regular FIT screening if FIT is negative. Every step may affect the screening effectiveness and the quality of screening programs may be jeopardized should any step is not taken carefully. For example, prolonged waiting time for colonoscopy may not only increase the risk of CRC and CRC death (Corley et al. 2014; Lee et al. 2019; Beshara et al. 2020), according to recent studies, but also affect the compliance with colonoscopy, leading to subsequent interval CRC (Jen et al. 2019). Dedicated call center may help this and intensify the proper screening process though additional manpower but well-training is needed.

Regional certified FIT laboratories may facilitate timely high-throughput management of stool samples in large administrative areas. In the Taiwanese screening program, some laboratories provide outreach services for collecting stool samples, and therefore diminish geographic or access barriers of the people, which largely contributes to increased screening uptake.

2.5.6 Information System

Health information systems required for a population-based organized service screening should have two basic functions: primary database system and linkage with external data sources. The primary database system consists of registration and data entry system, referral and follow-up system, and evaluation system. The detailed process has been elucidated in full elsewhere (Chiu et al. 2006). The unit of data entry is not only based on record but also take an individual or even family or pedigree into account. The data registration system not only considers the avoidance of unnecessary duplicate key-in procedure for health insurance payments after the out-reaching service transportation also reduces the possibility of shopping for health check-ups at different primary care units. Referral and follow-up systems are very flexible to recall attendees who have been informed to be requested for further confirmation of disease status. The system sometimes should be adapted to the setting patients are scheduled to be referred to or centrally regulated by the health center. Health information systems for screening should also include the evaluation of screening programs. External data linkage includes population registry, cancer and death registries, and claimed data on national health insurance.

2.5.7 Evidence-Based Evaluation

Evaluation of outcomes, especially its effectiveness is of utmost importance for a screening program. Distinct from a randomized trial, evaluation of service screening program is more complex and requires sophisticated methodological approaches because it is usually associated with confounding factors and biases, which need to be adjusted. Moreover, economic appraisal is another important aspect. It includes the selection of the strategy with lowest cost to achieve the maximum effectiveness (cost-effectiveness/utility analysis) and the assessment of whether and how much benefit could be accrued (cost-benefit analysis). Collaboration with academia can facilitate such process by the discovery of solution, knowledge transfer, and the enhancement of partnership. Some important screening quality indicators pertaining to important clinical outcomes (i.e., CRC death or incidence) could also be developed via such collaboration.

In summary, in order to fit in with evidence-based principle of screening, a well-organized service screening for CRC rather than opportunistic case-finding should be considered with the following components: (1) well-defined detection modes of early and late detection of cancers, age range, and inter-screening intervals, (2) organized referral and confirmatory diagnosis logistics, sufficient capacity of health care service (including management of neoplasm and clinical surveillance); (3) explicit quality metrics and monitoring/audit system; (4) comprehensive health information system dedicated for screening service; and (5) evidence-based evaluation including effectiveness or cost-effectiveness or cost-utility analysis.

References

Abu-Freha N. Should colonoscopy be the primary screening modality for colorectal cancer in Israel? Harefuah. 2019;158(8):523–8.

Association of European Cancer Leagues – Cancer Prevention. n.d.. https://www.europeancancerleagues.org/cancer-screening-in-europe/

Australian National Bowel Cancer Screening Program. n.d.. http://www.cancerscreening.gov.au/internet/screening/publishing.nsf/Content/bowel-screening-1

Belgium Colon Cancer Screening. n.d.. https://www.ddg-gastro.be/en/colon-cancer-screening/

Benson VS, Patnick J, Davies AK, Nadel MR, Smith RA, Atkin WS, International Colorectal Cancer Screening Network. Colorectal cancer screening: a comparison of 35 initiatives in 17 countries. Int J Cancer. 2008;122(6):1357–67.

Beshara A, Ahoroni M, Comanester D, et al. Association between time to colonoscopy after a positive guaiac fecal test result and risk of colorectal cancer and advanced stage disease at diagnosis. Int J Cancer. 2020;146(6):1532–40.

Boguradzka A, Wiszniewski M, Kaminski MF, Kraszewska E, Mazurczak-Pluta T, Rzewuska D, Ptasinski A, Regula J. The effect of primary care physician counseling on participation rate and use of sedation in colonoscopy-based colorectal cancer screening program–a randomized controlled study. Scand J Gastroenterol. 2014;49(7):878–84.

Bowel cancer screening, International Agency for Research on Cancer, WHO. n.d.. http://cancer-code-europe.iarc.fr/index.php/en/ecac-12-ways/screening-recommandation/bowel-cancer-screening

Bowel Screening. NHS Health Scotland. n.d.. https://www.nhsinform.scot/healthy-living/screening/bowel/bowel-screening

Bugajski M, Rupinski M, Wieszczy P, Pisera M, Regula J, Kaminski MF. Key performance measures for colonoscopy in the polish colonoscopy screening program. Endoscopy. 2019;51(09):858–65.

Cai SR, Zhang SZ, Zhu HH, Zheng S. Barriers to colorectal cancer screening: a case-control study. World J Gastroenterol. 2009;15(20):2531.

Cai SR, Huang YQ, Zhang SZ, Li QL, Ma XY, Zheng S. Effects of subitems in the colorectal cancer screening protocol on the Chinese colorectal cancer screening program: an analysis based on natural community screening results. BMC Cancer. 2019;19(1):47.

Canadian Cancer Society – Screening for Colorectal Cancer. n.d.. https://www.cancer.ca/en/cancer-information/cancer-type/colorectal/screening/?region=on

Cancer Control Act. Taiwan. 2003. https://www.hpa.gov.tw/Pages/Detail.aspx?nodeid=1057&pid=6023

Chiu YH, Chen LS, Chan CC, Liou DM, Wu SC, Kuo HS, Chang HJ, Chen TH. Health information system for community-based multiple screening in Keelung, Taiwan (Keelung community-based integrated Screening no. 3). Int J Med Inform. 2006;75(5):369–83.

Chiu HM, Chen SL, Yen AM, Chiu SY, Fann JC, Lee YC, Pan SL, Wu MS, Liao CS, Chen HH, Koong SL, Chiou ST. Effectiveness of fecal immunochemical testing in reducing colorectal cancer mortality from the one million Taiwanese Screening program. Cancer. 2015;121(18):3221–9.

Chiu HM, Hsu WF, Chang LC, Wu MH. Colorectal cancer screening in Asia. Curr Gastroenterol Rep. 2017;19(10):47.

Choi KS, Lee HY, Jun JK, Shin A, Park EC. Adherence to follow-up after a positive fecal occult blood test in an organized colorectal cancer screening program in Korea, 2004–2008. J Gastroenterol Hepatol. 2012;27(6):1070–7.

Chou CK, Chen SL, Yen AM, et al. Outreach and inreach organized service Screening programs for colorectal Cancer. PLoS One. 2016;11(5):e0155276.

Cole SR, Smith A, Wilson C, Turnbull D, Esterman A, Young GP. An advance notification letter increases participation in colorectal cancer screening. J Med Screen. 2007;14(2):73–5.

Colorectal Cancer Screening Programme, Ministry of Health, Welfare and Sport, the Netherlands. n.d.. https://www.rivm.nl/en/colorectal-cancer-screening-programme

Corley DA, Levin TR, Doubeni CA. Adenoma detection rate and risk of colorectal cancer and death. N Engl J Med. 2014;370(26):2541.

Courtier R, Casamitjana M, Macià F, Panadés A, Castells X, Gil MJ, Hidalgo JM, Sánchez-Ortega JM. Participation in a colorectal cancer screening programme: influence of the method of contacting the target population. Eur J Cancer Prev. 2002;11(3):209–13.

Department of Health – Prevent Colorectal Cancer (Hong Kong). n.d.. https://www.colonscreen.gov.hk/en/public/index.html

Digby J, McDonald PJ, Strachan JA, Libby G, Steele RJ, Fraser CG. Use of a faecal immunochemical test narrows current gaps in uptake for sex, age and deprivation in a bowel cancer screening programme. J Med Screen. 2013;20(2):80–5.

Division of Cancer Prevention and Control, Centers for Disease Control and Prevention, United States. n.d.. https://www.cdc.gov/cancer/crccp/index.htm

Dubé C. Organized screening is better than opportunistic Screening at decreasing the burden of colorectal cancer in the United States. Gastroenterology. 2018;155(5):1302–4.

European Colorectal Cancer Screening Guidelines Working Group, von Karsa L, Patnick J, Segnan N, Atkin W, Halloran S, et al. European guidelines for quality assurance in colorectal cancer screening and diagnosis: overview and introduction to the full supplement publication. Endoscopy. 2013;45(1):51–9. https://doi.org/10.1055/s-0032-1325997.

Forbes GM, Mendelson RM, Edwards JT, Foster NM, Pawlik JZ, Bampton PA, et al. A comparison of colorectal neoplasia screening tests: a multicentre community-based study of the impact of consumer choice. Med J Aust. 2006;184(11):546–50.

Giorgi Rossi P, Grazzini G, Anti M, Baiocchi D, Barca A, Bellardini P, Brezzi S, Camilloni L, Falini P, Maccallini V, Mantellini P, Romeo D, Rubeca T, Venditti MA. Direct mailing of faecal occult blood tests for colorectal cancer screening: a randomized population study from Central Italy. J Med Screen. 2011;18(3):121–7.

Hardcastle JD, Chamberlain JO, Robinson MH, et al. Randomised controlled trial of faecal-occult-blood screening for colorectal cancer. Lancet. 1996;348:1472–7.

Health Promotion Administration, 1e, Taiwan. n.d.. https://www.hpa.gov.tw/EngPages/Detail.aspx?nodeid=1051&pid=5957

Jen HH, Wang TH, Chiu HM, Peng SM, Hsu CY, Chiu SY, Chen SL, Yen AM, Lee YC, Chen HH, Fann JC. Hurdle Poisson regression model for identifying factors related to noncompliance and waiting time for confirmatory diagnosis in colorectal cancer screening. Int J Technol Assess Health Care. 2019;35(2):85–91.

Joseph DA, Meester RG, Zauber AG, Manninen DL, Winges L, Dong FB, Peaker B, van Ballegooijen M. Colorectal cancer screening: estimated future colonoscopy need and current volume and capacity. Cancer. 2016;122(16):2479–86.

Kaminski MF, Kraszewska E, Rupinski M, Laskowska M, Wieszczy P, Regula J. Design of the polish colonoscopy screening program: a randomized health services study. Endoscopy. 2015;47(12):1144–50.

Katičić M, Antoljak N, Kujundžić M, Stamenić V, Poljak DS, Kramarić D, Štimac D, Pešikan MS, Šamija M, Ebling Z. Results of national colorectal cancer screening program in Croatia (2007-2011). World J Gastroenterol: WJG. 2012;18(32):4300.

Kronborg O, Fenger C, Olsen J, Jorgensen OD, Sondergaard O. Randomised study of screening for colorectal cancer with faecal-occult-blood test. Lancet. 1996;348:1467–71.

Lee YC, Fann JC, Chiang TH, et al. Time to colonoscopy and risk of colorectal cancer in patients with positive results from fecal immunochemical tests. Clin Gastroenterol Hepatol. 2019;17(7):1332–40.

Levi Z, Birkenfeld S, Vilkin A, Bar-Chana M, Lifshitz I, Chared M, Maoz E, Niv Y. A higher detection rate for colorectal cancer and advanced adenomatous polyp for screening with immunochemical fecal occult blood test than guaiac fecal occult blood test, despite lower compliance rate. A prospective, controlled, feasibility study. Int J Cancer. 2011;128(10):2415–24.

Libby G, Bray J, Champion J, Brownlee LA, Birrell J, Gorman DR, Crighton EM, Fraser CG, Steele RJ. Prenotification increases uptake of colorectal cancer screening in all demographic groups: a randomized controlled trial. J Med Screen. 2011;18(1):24–9.

Mandel JS, Bond JH, Church TR, Snover DC, Bradley GM, Schuman LM, Ederer F. Reducing mortality from colorectal cancer by screening for fecal occult blood. Minnesota Colon Cancer control study. N Engl J Med. 1993;328(19):1365–71.

Ministry of Health, Labour and Welfare, Japan. n.d.. https://www.mhlw.go.jp/stf/seisakunitsuite/bunya/0000059490.html

Navarro M, Nicolas A, Ferrandez A, Lanas A. Colorectal cancer population screening programs worldwide in 2016: an update. World J Gastroenterol. 2017;23(20):3632.

NHS bowel cancer screening (BCSP) programme, United Kingdom. n.d.. https://www.gov.uk/topic/population-screening-programmes/bowel

Nnoaham KE, Lines C. Modelling future capacity needs and spending on colonoscopy in the English bowel cancer screening programme. Gut. 2008;57(9):1238–45.

Onyoh EF, Hsu WF, Chang LC, Lee YC, Wu MS, Chiu HM. The rise of colorectal cancer in Asia: epidemiology, screening, and management. Curr Gastroenterol Rep. 2019;21(8):36.

Poskus T, Strupas K, Mikalauskas S, Bitinaitė D, Kavaliauskas A, Samalavicius NE, Saladzinskas

Z. Initial results of the national colorectal cancer screening program in Lithuania. Eur J Cancer Prev. 2015;24(2):76–80.

Rabeneck L. Colorectal cancer screening: opportunistic or organized? Can J Gastroenterol. 2006;20(4):249–50.

Rabeneck L, Chiu HM, Senore C. International perspective on the burden of colorectal Cancer and public health effects. Gastroenterology. 2020;158(2):447–52.

Sanduleanu S, le Clercq CM, Dekker E, et al. Definition and taxonomy of interval colorectal cancers: a proposal for standardising nomenclature. Gut. 2015;64(8):1257–67.

Sano Y, Byeon JS, Li XB, Wong MC, Chiu HM, Rerknimitr R, Utsumi T, Hattori S, Sano W, Iwatate M, Chiu P, Sung J. Colorectal cancer screening of the general population in East Asia. Dig Endosc. 2016;28(3):243–9.

Santé Publique France – National colo rectal cancer screening programme. France. n.d.. https://www.santepubliquefrance.fr/maladies-et-traumatismes/cancers/cancer-du-colon-rectum/documents/communication-congres/national-colo-rectal-cancer-screening-programme-france

Schreuders EH, Ruco A, Rabeneck L, Schoen RE, Sung JJ, Young GP, Kuipers EJ. Colorectal cancer screening: a global overview of existing programmes. Gut. 2015;64(10):1637–49.

Scottish Bowel Screening Programme, Public Health Scotland. n.d.. https://www.isdscotland.org/Health-Topics/Cancer/Bowel-Screening/

Seeff LC, Manninen DL, Dong FB, Chattopadhyay SK, Nadel MR, Tangka FK, Molinari NA. Is there endoscopic capacity to provide colorectal cancer screening to the unscreened population in the United States? Gastroenterology. 2004;127(6):1661–9.

Senore C, Inadomi J, Segnan N, Bellisario C, Hassan C. Optimising colorectal cancer screening acceptance: a review. Gut. 2015;64(7):1158–77.

Strnad M, Šogorić S. Rano otkrivanje raka u Hrvatskoj. Acta Medica Croatica. 2014;64(5):461–7.

Suchanek S, Majek O, Vojtechova G, Minarikova P, Rotnaglova B, Seifert B, Minarik M, Kozeny P, Dusek L, Zavoral M. Colorectal cancer prevention in the Czech Republic: time trends in performance indicators and current situation after 10 years of screening. Eur J Cancer Prev. 2014;23(1):18–26.

Swan H, Siddiqui AA, Myers RE. International colorectal cancer screening programs: population contact strategies, testing methods and screening rates. Pract Gastroenterol. 2012;36(8):20–9.

The Reference Centre for Epidemiology and Cancer Prevention in Piemonte, Italy. n.d.. https://www.cpo.it/en/data/screening/

Tinmouth J, Patel J, Austin PC, Baxter NN, Brouwers MC, Earle C, Levitt C, Lu Y, Mackinnon M, Paszat L, Rabeneck L. Increasing participation in colorectal cancer screening: results from a cluster randomized trial of directly mailed g FOBT kits to previous non-responders. Int J Cancer. 2015;136(6):E697–703.

Van Roosbroeck S, Hoeck S, Van Hal G. Population-based screening for colorectal cancer using an immunochemical faecal occult blood test: a comparison of two invitation strategies. Cancer Epidemiol. 2012;36(5):e317–24.

Options of Colorectal Cancer Screening: An Overview

Tsung-Hsien Chiang and Yi-Chia Lee

Abstract

Colorectal cancer is not only a significant health issue in industrialized and developed countries; its incidence rate is also increasing in developing countries, making it the most prevalent cancer on a global scale. Given the limited effect of risk factor modification for primary prevention, secondary prevention—in the form of screening and early detection—is currently the most effective approach to reducing deaths from colorectal cancer through the use of colonoscopy. Nonetheless, colonoscopy itself is time-consuming, labor-intensive, and not without risk; also, the resource constraint of the limited number of endoscopists makes it not practical to serve as the primary screening tool in many countries. To enable better resource allocation, a two-stage approach is increasingly popular: first, a noninvasive screening test, then a confirmatory examination such as colonoscopy. Such an approach has two advantages: a higher participation rate when most of the target population is asymptomatic and better resource allocation when the screening test is highly accurate in identifying subjects with colorectal neoplasms. Several types of screening tests are available, including stool-based tests, such as the guaiac-based fecal occult blood test, the fecal immunochemical test, and the stool DNA test, and blood-based tests, such as the plasmic methylated septin-9 test. Even for the image-based tests, there are noninvasive tests, such as the computed tomographic colonography and colon capsule endoscopy, in addition to the invasive studies of flexible sigmoidoscopy and colonoscopy. Here, we present a precis of the performance and clinical application of these tests for mass screening.

T.-H. Chiang
Department of Internal Medicine, College of Medicine, National Taiwan University, Taipei, Taiwan

Department of Integrated Diagnostics and Therapeutics, National Taiwan University Hospital, Taipei, Taiwan

Graduate Institute of Clinical Medicine, College of Medicine, National Taiwan University, Taipei, Taiwan

Y.-C. Lee (✉)
Department of Internal Medicine, College of Medicine, National Taiwan University, Taipei, Taiwan

Graduate Institute of Epidemiology and Preventive Medicine, College of Public Health, National Taiwan University, Taipei, Taiwan
e-mail: yichialee@ntu.edu.tw

Keywords

Colorectal cancer screening · Guaiac-based fecal occult blood test · Fecal immunochemical test · Fecal hemoglobin concentration Stool DNA test · Fecal microbiota · Plasmic methylated septin-9 · Computed tomographic colonography · Colon capsule endoscopy Flexible sigmoidoscopy · Colonoscopy

© Springer Nature Singapore Pte Ltd. 2021
H.-M. Chiu, H.-H. Chen (eds.), *Colorectal Cancer Screening*,
https://doi.org/10.1007/978-981-15-7482-5_3

3.1   Introduction

Given the rapid increase in the incidence rate due to the Westernization of lifestyle, colorectal cancer (CRC) poses a significant threat to global health as the second and third most common cause of cancer-related death in men and women, respectively (Siegel et al. 2017; Bishehsari et al. 2014). Although international guidelines and expert consensus have recommended CRC screening for asymptomatic individuals aged 50 years or more (Benard et al. 2018), an increasing trend of CRC risk is generally observed recently in younger generations (Lee et al. 2019a). Given the foreseeable increase in disease burden, an effective strategy to eliminate the threat from CRC is urgently needed (Inra and Syngal 2015; Chiu et al. 2015).

Cancer stage at diagnosis is the most crucial determinant of the survival rate. To reach the goal of early diagnosis, colonoscopy can identify superficial cancerous foci to reduce the rate of CRC-related death, and also offers an opportunity to remove the precancerous lesions (adenomatous polyps) to reduce the number of newly developed cases. However, it still represents a challenge as a primary screening tool due to the limited number of certified endoscopists in most countries (Rex and Lieberman 2001). Therefore, risk stratification is needed for the asymptomatic populations in order to better allocate endoscopy resources (Chiu et al. 2016). In the first stage, noninvasive test with good sensitivity and specificity to detect CRC or advanced adenomas will increase the uptake or adherence rate of asymptomatic populations to screening. In the subsequent second stage for those with positive results, it would increase the colonoscopic yield rate in the discovery of early-stage neoplasms, and potentially make the screening program more cost-effective. Nowadays, the noninvasive triage screening tests that commercially available for screening can be categorized into the stool-based tests and the blood-based tests (Fig. 3.1). The former includes the guaiac fecal occult blood test (gFOBT), the fecal immunochemical test (FIT), and the stool DNA test, while the latter include the plasmic methylated septin-9 test (*SEPT9*). In addition, we will also introduce the direct visualizing screening or diagnostic modalities, including computed tomographic colonography (CTC), colon capsule endoscopy (CCE), flexible sigmoidoscopy, and colonoscopy (Fig. 3.1). In this chapter, we

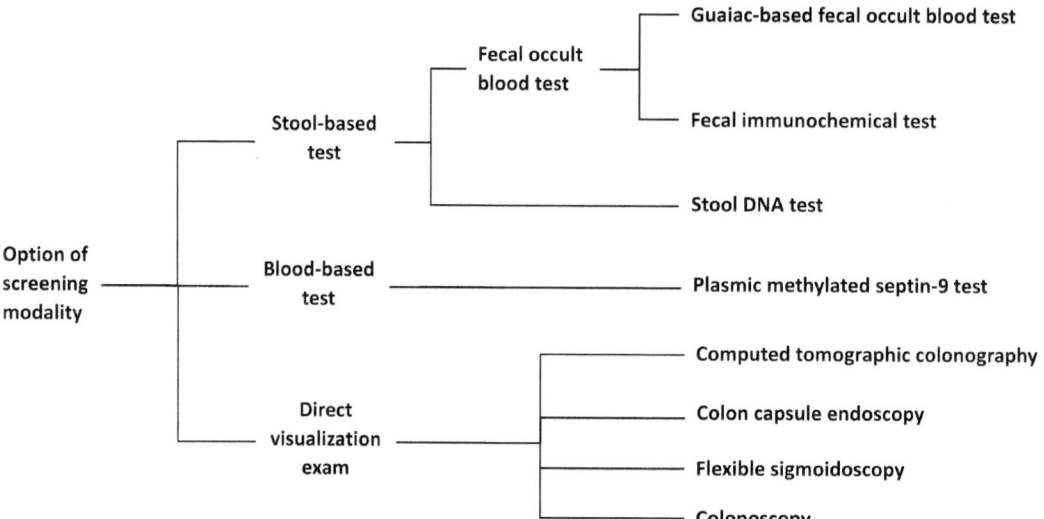

Fig. 3.1 Option of colorectal cancer screening modalities. Stool-based tests include guaiac fecal occult blood test, fecal immunochemical test, and stool DNA test. Blood-based test is a plasmic methylated septin-9 test.

Direct visualization examinations include computed tomographic colonography, colon capsule endoscopy, flexible sigmoidoscopy, and colonoscopy

will address the performance of these tests and compare their merits and drawbacks in the context of mass screening. We will also discuss the emerging roles of measuring the hemoglobin concentration in the stool sample for precise risk stratification and the possibility of quantifying the gut microbiota dysbiosis, for both the primary and the secondary prevention of CRC.

3.2   Stool-Based Tests for Screening

3.2.1   The Fecal Occult Blood Test

When a colorectal tumor increases in size and invasiveness, it starts to shed measurable blood into the feces. The guaiac-based method of detecting occult blood in the feces is the most traditional approach for CRC screening. It involves placing stool samples on the guaiac paper to detect the hemoglobin in feces through the chemical reaction between the heme and the guaiac. Using the gFOBT (for example, the Hemoccult SENSA), previous researchers have demonstrated sensitivity of 79.4% (95% confidence interval [CI]: 64.3–94.5%) and specificity of 86.7% (95% CI: 85.9–87.4%) to detect CRC (Allison et al. 1996). One drawback of this approach is the need for dietary restriction to avoid false-positive results from iron supplements, red meat containing non-human hemoglobin, and certain vegetables containing chemicals with peroxidase properties (Rockey 1999). Another drawback is related to the limited ability of this test to differentiate between the blood spilled from the upper gastrointestinal tract and that from the lower gastrointestinal tract (Chiang et al. 2011). Furthermore, the judgment of positivity is rather subjective, and the need for trained personnel to visually interpret the test results also constrains its application for mass screening.

By contrast, the FIT is specific for human globin (Carroll et al. 2014). A study using an asymptomatic cohort of 2796 subjects who received same-day upper and lower endoscopic examinations demonstrated that FIT was specific for predicting lesions in the lower gastrointestinal tract but unable to detect lesions in the upper gastrointestinal tract (Chiang et al. 2011). Besides, the prevalence rate of lesions in the upper gastrointestinal tract did not differ significantly between subjects with positive and negative FIT results. Another significant advantage of FIT is its ability to provide both qualitative and quantitative measures of the hemoglobin concentration. The former, the qualitative FIT, uses the lateral flow immune-chromatographic method so it can, similar to the guaiac-based test, rapidly provide a visualized result when the concentration of hemoglobin in feces is higher than the cutoff value defined by the manufacturer (Hundt et al. 2009). The quantitative FIT uses the immune-turbidimetric method to measure the hemoglobin concentration in the stool sample. Even though both approaches are based on the same mechanism of an antibody–antigen reaction, the quantitative FIT additionally provides a numerical measure so that the cutoff value for a positive result can be adjusted according to the tradeoff between the number of colonoscopies needed and the colonoscopy yield rate of neoplasms.

In terms of test performance, the simultaneous uses of colonoscopy and qualitative FIT (OC-Light (V-PC50 and V-PH80); Eiken Chemical Co. Ltd., Tokyo, Japan) in a hospital-based study showed a sensitivity of 78.6% (95% CI: 58.5–91.0%) and specificity of 92.8% (95% CI: 92.5–93.2%), for the detection of CRC with the cutoff value of 10 μg Hb/g feces (Chiu et al. 2013). Similarly, one pooled analysis that included nine studies from different ethnic populations found a sensitivity of 89% (95% CI: 80–95%) and specificity of 91% (95% CI: 89–93%) in detecting CRC with a cutoff value of 20 μg Hb/g feces (Lee et al. 2014). Although no randomized controlled trials have yet demonstrated that FIT is superior to gFOBT in terms of the final endpoint of CRC mortality rate, one meta-analysis of 14 randomized controlled trials did compare the performance of FIT with that of gFOBT, finding that FIT could detect more than twice as many CRCs (2.28-fold; 95% CI: 1.68–3.10) and advanced adenomas than gFOBT (Hassan et al. 2012). In addition to its better test performance, FIT also has the advantage of using a rapid, mass throughput system to cope with a large number of returned samples, making it increasingly popular in clinical practice and especially widely used for large-scale population screening programs (Zhu et al. 2010; Tinmouth et al. 2015).

One potential problem of the quantitative FIT is the difficulty of comparing numerical test results between different products. Since the antibodies used to detect hemoglobin, the buffer, and the sampling device may vary, different brands of quantitative FIT, even those which claim the same cutoff value, can still differ in terms of test performance. In a nationwide study in Taiwan, two quantitative FITs (OC-Sensor and HM-Jack) with the same cutoff concentration of 20 μg Hb/g feces demonstrated different performance, especially in the ability to detect proximally located CRCs (Chiang et al. 2014). In a randomized trial from the Netherlands, two quantitative FITs (OC-Sensor and FOB-Gold) with the same cutoff concentration of 10 μg Hb/g feces also showed different positivity rates and led to different diagnostic yields (Grobbee et al. 2017).

Most of the quantitative FITs give the cutoff concentration as ng Hb/mL buffer. Because different brands of FIT have different devices in the sampling stick and different volumes of buffer, it is difficult to compare the results from different brands of FIT. To solve this problem, a standardized system of FIT results has been proposed, with a unified measure of μg Hb/g feces. With this unified unit, it makes the results from different quantitative FITs more comparable (Chiang et al. 2014).

3.2.2 The Role of Fecal Hemoglobin Concentration

Recently, researches indicated that the quantitative measure of fecal hemoglobin concentration (FHbC) is a useful indicator for both the risk stratification for CRC and the priority setting of colonoscopy. One population-based study from Taiwan has shown that a baseline FIT concentration even lower than the cutoff value considered a positive result (i.e., 20 μg Hb/g feces) was

associated with a subsequent risk of colorectal neoplasia during the longitudinal follow-up (Chen et al. 2011). Besides, in those with a positive FIT result (higher than the cutoff value of 20 μg Hb/g feces) who did not receive a diagnostic colonoscopy, a higher FHbC at baseline was associated with an increased risk of death from CRC. A gradient relationship was seen: the risk of death was 1.31-fold (95% CI: 1.04–1.71), 2.21-fold (95% CI: 1.55–3.34), and 2.53-fold (95% CI: 1.95–3.43), respectively, for subjects with FHbC of 20–49, 50–99, and >100 μg Hb/g feces, respectively, who did not receive colonoscopic follow-up, as compared with similar subjects with colonoscopic follow-up (Lee et al. 2017). The wait time for a colonoscopy after a positive result of FIT was also associated with increased risk. A significantly gradient relationship was seen between the quantitative value of FIT at baseline and the subsequent risk of any CRC and advanced-stage disease (Lee et al. 2019b). Using patients with a fecal hemoglobin concentration of 20–49 μg Hb/g feces as the baseline, each increase of 10 μg Hb/g feces was associated with a 9.9% greater risk of CRC (95% CI: 9.4–10.5%) and a 12.7% greater risk of advanced-stage disease (95% CI: 11.5–13.9%) (Lee et al. 2019b).

3.2.3 Stool DNA Test

The development of CRC is associated with the progression and accumulation of genetic and epigenetic damage, resulting in the inactivation of tumor suppressor genes and activation of the oncogene. Therefore, the direct detection of abnormal DNAs or epigenetic markers shed from colorectal neoplasms into the feces becomes a valuable approach. The commercially available stool DNA test mainly detects DNA mutations, microsatellite instability, impaired DNA mismatch repair, and abnormal DNA methylation. A pilot study of such testing with a panel of 15 point mutations of K-RAS, p-53, APC, and BAT-26 (a microsatellite instability marker) showed a sensitivity of 91% for CRC and 82% for adenomas ≥1 cm, with a specificity of 93% (Ahlquist et al.

2000). In an US large-scale study, 9899 asymptomatic individuals aged 50–84 years underwent testing with the multitarget stool DNA panel, including K-RAS point mutations, aberrantly methylated NDRG4 and BMP3, the β-actin gene (to serve as a control indicator of DNA quantity), with FIT as the reference standard. The results showed that the stool DNA panel had a higher sensitivity of 92.3% for CRC, compared to 73.8% for FIT, and a higher sensitivity of 42.4% for advanced precancerous lesions (advanced adenoma or sessile serrated polyp ≥1 cm), compared to 23.8% for FIT; nonetheless, specificity for stool DNA testing was lower at 86.6% (Imperiale et al. 2014). The multitarget stool DNA panel combines various detecting technologies to detect CRC and early colorectal lesions with higher sensitivity; the weakness, however, in terms of the wide application of this panel, is its very higher cost and lower specificity.

3.2.4 Fecal Microbiota as a Potential Biomarker for CRC Screening

Although the role of the gut microbiota in CRC is currently under enthusiastic exploration, there is limited information on the real-world application for CRC screening. One study found that increased CRC risk was associated with decreased bacterial diversity in feces, depletion of Gram-positive, fiber-fermenting Clostridia, and increased presence of the Gram-negative, pro-inflammatory genera *Fusobacterium* and *Porphyromonas* (Ahn et al. 2013). One retrospective case-control study, which evaluated the performance of FIT combined with microbial markers to screen for CRC and advanced adenoma, showed that combining FIT with quantitative fecal *Fusobacterium nucleatum* significantly increased the detection rates for CRC, with a sensitivity of 92.3% and specificity of 93.0%; for advanced adenoma, the results were 38.6% and 89.0%, respectively, providing additional information for a FIT-based screening program (Wong et al. 2017). Although longitudinal studies are required to further assess the predictive value of microbiota as a biomarker, the topic

represents a novel and promising approach (Gagniere et al. 2016).

3.3 Blood-Based Tests for Screening

3.3.1 Plasmic Methylated Septin-9

Carcinoembryonic antigen is the common serum-based glycoprotein CRC marker used in monitoring disease recurrence or the response to therapy and in predicting prognosis; however, it is not recommended for CRC screening due to low sensitivity and the lack of CRC specificity, especially for early-stage CRC (Locker et al. 2006). Instead, the methylation of the *SEPT9* gene, a tumor suppressor gene, has been identified by comparing multiple candidate markers in normal colonic epithelium and CRC tissue samples (Lofton-Day et al. 2008). The blood-based *SEPT9* gene methylation assay thus aims to detect the aberrant methylation at the promoter region of the *SEPT9* gene DNA released from CRC cells into the peripheral blood (Lofton-Day et al. 2008). Reports on the *SEPT9* assay used the 1/3, 2/3, 1/2, or 1/1 algorithm to define a positive test, depending on the number of PCR assays (the denominator) performed and the number of positive PCR reactions (the numerator) (Song et al. 2017). In one multicenter study using colonoscopy as a reference standard, the researchers investigated the application of this blood test to detect asymptomatic CRC in an average-risk population; the results showed a sensitivity of 48.2% and 63.9% and a specificity of 91.5% and 88.4% using an 1/2 or 1/3 algorithm, respectively; however, the sensitivity for advanced adenoma was low at 11.2% (Church et al. 2014). According to the pooled data in the meta-analysis, the *SEPT9* assay had higher sensitivity than the FIT test (75.6% vs. 67.1%) while the specificity was similar (90.4% vs. 92.0%) in a symptomatic population; in contrast, the *SEPT9* assay exhibited lower sensitivity (68.0% vs. 79.0%) and lower specificity (80.0% vs. 94.0%) than the FIT test in an asymptomatic population (Song et al. 2017). The results may indicate different capabilities in detecting early-stage neoplasms, which may require further evaluation. Owing to its insufficient sensitivity to detect early-stage CRC or advanced adenoma, though being approved by the US FDA, such test is recommended to be used for screening only if the screening subjects were not compliant to currently recommended screening test like FIT, gFOBT, endoscopic (colonoscopy or flexible sigmoidoscopy), or CTC screening (Rex et al. 2017).

Though there are several blood biomarkers developed for detecting CRC, only a few had tested their performance in the real screening population regarding screening uptake, neoplasm detection, and effectiveness (Elshimali et al. 2013; Gezer et al. 2015). Further studies in a screening setting are required before their use as the frontline CRC screening tests.

3.4 Estimation of CRC Risk Based on Screening Test Results

The performance of clinically available screening modalities using colonoscopy as the reference standard for CRC and advanced colorectal neoplasms are summarized in Tables 3.1 and 3.2, respectively. As demonstrated in Fig. 3.2, the posttest probability of disease can be estimated by using the base-line risk of an individual and the result of a screening test. For example, in subjects at average risk of CRC, one may expect a prevalence rate of 0.1% for CRC; given a positive FIT result, the posttest probability can be increased to 1% (0.1% × positive likelihood ratio of 10). Therefore, colonoscopic follow-up is recommended. By contrast, the posttest probability can be lowered as far as to 0.01% (0.1% × negative likelihood ratio of 0.1) with a negative result of a stool DNA test, which suggests that such subjects do not need a colonoscopy. Therefore, in clinical practice, different tests may have different advantages in ruling in or ruling out subjects by CRC risk.

3.5 Direct Visualizing Examinations for CRC Screening

3.5.1 Double-Contrast Barium Enema

In double-contrast barium enema (DCBE), the colon is studied through X-rays obtained after coating the mucosa with barium and distending the colon with air via transrectal insertion. In a

Table 3.1 Performance of available clinical screening modalities for colorectal cancer using colonoscopy as a reference standard

Screening modality	Sensitivity, % (95% CI)	Specificity, % (95% CI)	Positive likelihood ratio (95% CI)	Negative likelihood ratio (95% CI)
Fecal-based test				
gFOBT (Allison et al. 1996)	79.4 (64.3–94.5)	86.7 (85.9–87.4)	5.98 (4.27–8.37)	0.24 (0.17–0.33)
FIT (Chiu et al. 2013)	78.6 (58.5–91.0)	92.8 (92.5–93.2)	10.97 (7.58–15.90)	0.23 (0.16–0.33)
Multitarget stool DNA test (Imperiale et al. 2014)	92.3 (83.0–97.5)	86.6 (85.9–87.2)	5.90 (4.63–7.53)	0.09 (0.07–0.12)
Blood-based test				
Plasmic methylated septin-9 (Church et al. 2014)	48.2 (32.4–63.6)	91.5 (89.7–93.1)	5.89 (4.48–7.75)	0.54 (0.41–0.71)
Direct visualization examination				
Computed tomographic colonography (Johnson et al. 2008)	90 (84–96)	86 (81–90)	6.4 (5.7–7.2)	0.12 (0.07–0.20)
Colon capsule endoscopy (Van Gossum et al. 2009)	74 (52–88)	74 (72–75)	2.8	0.35
Flexible sigmoidoscopy (Niedermaier et al. 2018)[a]	79.3	–	–	–

CI confidence interval, *gFOBT* guaiac fecal occult blood test, *FIT* fecal immunochemical test
[a]Flexible sigmoidoscopy identified 169 distal colorectal cancers and missed 44 proximal colorectal cancers

Table 3.2 Performance of available clinical screening modalities for advanced colorectal neoplasms using colonoscopy as a reference standard

Screening modality	Sensitivity, % (95% CI)	Specificity, % (95% CI)	Positive likelihood ratio (95% CI)	Negative likelihood ratio (95% CI)
Fecal-based test				
gFOBT (Zhu et al. 2010)	54 (48–60)	80 (78–82)	2.7	0.58
FIT (Zhu et al. 2010)	67 (61–73)	85 (83–87)	4.5	0.39
Multitarget stool DNA test (Imperiale et al. 2014)	42.4 (38.9–46.0)	86.6 (85.9–87.3)	3.16 (2.93–3.40)	0.67 (0.72–0.62)
Blood-based test				
Plasmic methylated septin-9 (Church et al. 2014)	11.2 (7.2–15.7)	91.6 (89.9–93.1)	1.14 (1.00–1.29)	0.99 (0.87–1.12)
Direct visualization exam				
Computed tomographic colonography (Johnson et al. 2008)	90 (84–96)	86 (81–90)	6.4 (5.7–7.2)	0.12 (0.07–0.20)
Colon capsule endoscopy (Rex et al. 2015)	92 (82–97)	95 (93–97)	18.4	0.08
Flexible sigmoidoscopy (Khalid-de Bakker et al. 2011)[a]	73.7 (56.9–86.6)	89.3 (85.2–92.7)	6.9	0.29

CI confidence interval, *gFOBT* guaiac fecal occult blood test, *FIT* fecal immunochemical test
[a]The findings of flexible sigmoidoscopy were conducted from colonoscopy reports and defined as an examination of the distal colon

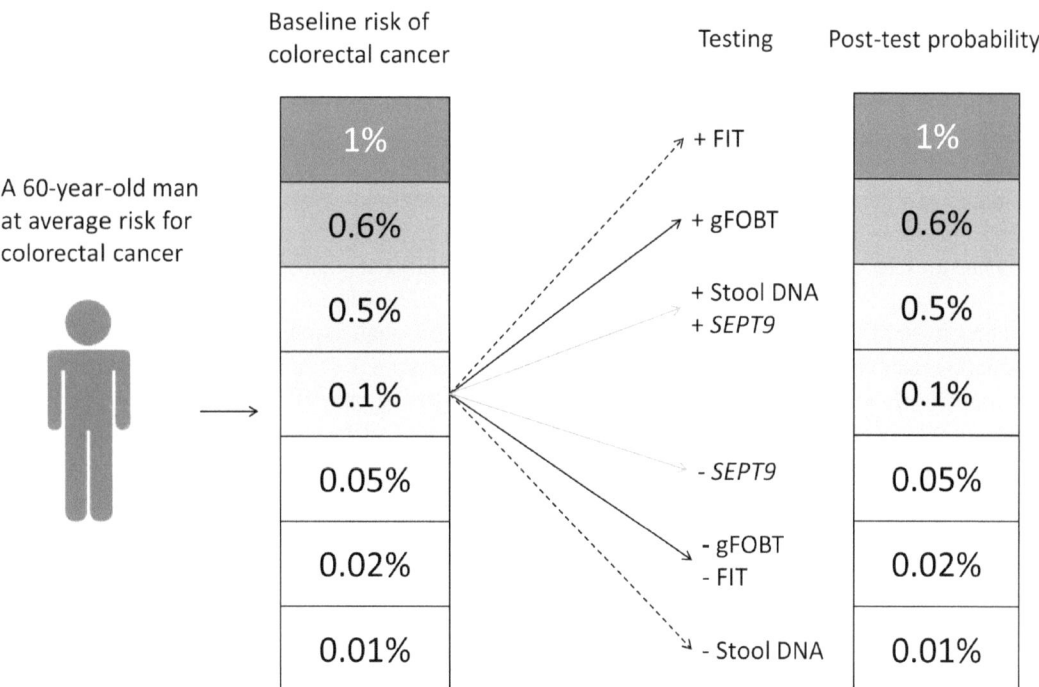

Fig. 3.2 Calculation of the posttest probability of an outcome by multiplying the baseline risk of an individual with the likelihood ratio of a positive or negative screening test result. We assume that the positive/negative likelihood ratios of guaiac fecal occult blood test (gFOBT), fecal immunochemical test (FIT), multitarget stool DNA test (stool DNA), and plasmic methylated septin-9 (*SEPT9*) are 6/0.2, 10/0.2, 5/0.1, and 5/0.5, respectively

comparison study, DCBE followed 7–14 days later by CTC and colonoscopy on the same day, the sensitivities of DCBE for lesions ≥10 mm and 6–9 mm were 48% and 35%, respectively (Rockey et al. 2005). Because of its low sensitivity, DCBE is not recommended as a first-line option for CRC screening (Sung et al. 2008).

3.5.2 Computed Tomographic Colonography

CTC uses advanced visualization technology and provides 2- or 3-dimensional endoluminal images of the colon upon reconstructing of computed tomography of the cleansed and air-distended colon (Kay and Evangelou 1996). It has several potential advantages over other screening tests for CRC, including relatively noninvasive technique, rapid imaging of the entire colon, no need for sedation, a low risk of procedure-related complications, and enabling review of extra-colonic organs in addition to the colonic mucosa (Pickhardt 2006). In one tandem study (a comparison study in which the same person was screened sequentially with same-day CTC and colonoscopy), the detection rates of advanced neoplasia (advanced adenoma or cancer) were similar with both screening methods; the sensitivity/specificity of CTC for the detection of adenomas or cancers were 65%/89% for lesions ≥5 mm and 90%/86% for lesions ≥10 mm (Johnson et al. 2008). In a randomized trial, detection rates with CTC, as compared with colonoscopy, were similar for CRC (0.5% vs. 0.5%) but were lower for all advanced adenomas (5.6% vs. 8.2%) and for advanced adenomas ≥10 mm (5.4% vs. 6.3%); besides, participation in this population-based screening program with CTC was significantly better than with colonoscopy (34% vs. 22%) (Stoop et al. 2012). Potential disadvantages associated with CTC include radiation exposure and requiring follow-up colonoscopy after positive results. Besides, CTC involves specially trained and qualified radiologists, which may not be comparable to most practice settings where few radiologists have access to similar training or technology. Generalizability of the findings to a community setting is limited because participating centers were large, academic institutions. Currently, there is limited evidence that a single screening with CTC reduces CRC incidence or mortality.

3.5.3 Colon Capsule Endoscopy

The first-generation colon capsule endoscopy (CCE-1) method for CRC screening was initially introduced in 2006, and consists of swallowing a pill-shaped device which is capable of photographing the gastrointestinal tract as it passes through it; however, low sensitivity but high specificity for detecting large polyps and advanced adenomas was demonstrated, and accuracy for detecting CRC was limited (Van Gossum et al. 2009). With the introduction of the second-generation CCE (CCE-2) in 2009 and the implementation of more standardized bowel cleansing protocols, the detection of colonic lesions has significantly increased diagnostic accuracy (Eliakim et al. 2009). In a prospective study for asymptomatic subjects who underwent CCE-2 followed by colonoscopy, the sensitivity and specificity of CCE-2 for detecting adenoma ≥6 mm was 88% (95% CI: 82–93%) and 82% (95% CI: 80–83%), respectively, and for detecting adenoma ≥10 mm were 92% (95% CI: 82–97%) and 95% (95% CI: 94–95%), respectively (Rex et al. 2015). Although CCE has shown to be a feasible and exceptionally safe procedure for the visualization of the entire colon, the overall accuracy of CCE largely depends on bowel cleanliness and still needs a referral to colonoscopy for clarification of detected lesion. Its high cost, requiring even more amount of bowel cleansing agent before capsule ingestion, and not being able to perform polypectomy are some of the constraints of this modality to be used as the primary screening modality.

3.5.4 Flexible Sigmoidoscopy

The flexible sigmoidoscopy provides visualization of the distal part of the large bowel up to the splenic flexure by using a flexible, 60-cm long endoscope. It requires only minimal bowel preparation and no sedation. It also provides the ability to excise or biopsy detected lesions during the same procedure. In a prospective study concerning the detection of advanced adenomas for an average-risk screening population who underwent sigmoidoscopy with colonoscopy as a reference standard, the sensitivity and specificity were 73.7% (95% CI: 56.9–86.6%) and 89.3% (95% CI: 85.2–92.7%), respectively (Khalid-de Bakker et al. 2011). One updated meta-analysis of randomized controlled trials estimated relative risks after screening with flexible sigmoidoscopy on CRC incidence and mortality were 0.82 (95% CI: 0.75–0.89) and 0.72 (95% CI: 0.65–0.80), respectively (Brenner et al. 2014). Its effectiveness is, however, only confined to distal colon and rectum, and the potential to detect proximal neoplasms depends on colonoscopy referral (Niedermaier et al. 2018).

3.5.5 Colonoscopy

The traditional method of colonoscopy provides visualization of the entire large bowel and the distal part of the small bowel by using a flexible, 130-cm to a 160-cm long endoscope. It is considered as the "gold standard" examination for CRC screening, mainly because of its high sensitivity and specificity for detecting not only cancerous but also precancerous lesions. It also provides the ability to excise or biopsy detected lesions during the same procedure. In the National Polyp Study, after 15 years follow-up, the standardized incidence-based mortality ratio was 0.47 (95% CI: 0.26–0.80) with colonoscopic polypectomy, suggesting a 53% reduction in mortality (Zauber et al. 2012). Although colonoscopy screening is recommended for the prevention of CRC in several European countries and the United States, no randomized trials so far have quantified its possible benefit. With colonoscopy as compared with no colonoscopy, one long-term observational study showed that hazard ratios for CRC were 0.57 (95% CI: 0.45–0.72) after polypectomy and 0.44 (95% CI: 0.38–0.52) after negative colonoscopy (Nishihara et al. 2013). One updated meta-analysis of observational studies estimated relative risks after

screening colonoscopy on CRC incidence and mortality were 0.31 (95% CI: 0.12–0.77) and 0.32 (95% CI: 0.23–0.43), respectively (Brenner et al. 2014). Although evidence shows that CRC screening with colonoscopy has the potential to prevent colorectal cancer of the entire large bowel, it is also associated with higher costs, complication rates, colonoscopist capacities, and not without risk.

3.6 Options for CRC Screening in Primary Care Setting

The advantages, disadvantages, and recommended interval of clinically available screening modalities for CRC are summarized in Table 3.3. There are significant differences in the adherence rates and participant preferences between colonoscopy and FIT according to the education, marital status, household income, and self-perceived risk of CRC (Wong et al. 2012). One American study has found that that primary colonoscopic screening might result in a lower completion rate as compared with the fecal occult blood testing; moreover, they also noted that there were differences in the racial/ethnic groups in the completion of fecal occult blood testing and colonoscopy (Inadomi et al. 2012). One Asian study showed that patients who were offered an informed choice (yearly FIT for up to 3 years or one-time colonoscopy) had higher adherence rates than patients who were not offered a choice, suggesting that providing a screening test option is of benefit (Wong et al. 2014). Although no trials have reported long-term findings of direct comparisons of the various screening modalities, the simulation studies have provided a way to extrapolate available evidence (Knudsen et al. 2016). In one simulation modeling study, assuming 100% adherence, the strategies of colonoscopy every 10 years, annual FIT, sigmoidoscopy every 10 years with annual FIT, and CTC every 5 years performed from ages 50 through 75 years can yield similar life-years gained, which indicate different individuals may consider different strategies for screening, in order to maximize the benefit (Knudsen et al. 2016).

Table 3.3 Summary of screening modalities in advantages, disadvantages, and recommended screening intervals

Screening modality	Advantages	Disadvantages	Recommended screening intervals
Fecal-based test			
Guaiac fecal occult blood test	No direct risk to colon; no bowel preparation; sampling at home; cheap	Miss polyps/cancer; false-positive result; colonoscopy needed if positive result; diet/medication restriction	Annual
Fecal immunochemical test	No direct risk to colon; no bowel preparation; sampling at home; no diet/medication restriction; cheap	Miss polyps/cancer; false-positive result; colonoscopy needed if positive result	Annual or biennial
Multitarget stool DNA test	No direct risk to colon; no bowel preparation; sampling at home; no diet/medication restriction	Miss polyps/cancer; false-positive result; colonoscopy needed if positive result; expensive	Every 3 years
Blood-based test			
Plasmic methylated septin-9 test	No direct risk to colon; no bowel preparation; no diet/medication restriction	Miss polyps/cancer; colonoscopy needed if positive result; expensive	Limited evidence
Direct visualization exam			
Computed tomographic colonography	No direct risk to colon; examine entire colon via virtual image	Bowel preparation; radiation exposure; false-positive result; colonoscopy needed if positive result; expensive	Every 5 years
Colon capsule endoscopy	No direct risk to colon; examine entire colon	Bowel preparation; colonoscopy needed if positive result; expensive	Every 5 years
Flexible sigmoidoscopy	Minimal bowel preparation; direct polyps/cancer sampling or resection; no conscious sedation; cheap	Examine distal colon; miss polyps/cancer; risk of bowel perforation and bleeding; colonoscopy needed if positive result	Every 5 years
Colonoscopy	Exam entire colon; direct polyps/cancer sampling or resection	Bowel preparation; risk of bowel perforation and bleeding; need conscious sedation; expensive	Every 10 years

3.7 Summary

CRC, historically a cancer typical of industrialized countries, is now a very common cancer and cause of cancer death globally. Evidence suggests that the disease is significantly increased in most developing countries, heralding an even greater disease burden in the near future. Colonoscopy remains the golden standard in diagnosis while a noninvasive test, using either fecal- or blood-based samples, or less invasive imaging tests, could be more suitable for population screening and provide guidance for individualized risk assessment prior to the invasive test of colonoscopy. The majority of guidelines recommend screening average-risk individuals aged 50–75 years using the fecal occult blood test

(mainly the FIT, annually or biennially), with quantitative FHbC of FIT serving as the population stratification tool for CRC risk prediction. The sensitivity of the stool DNA panel test is higher due to its combination of multiple detection points in feces. However, the high cost and lower specificity may need improvement before it can be widely used for population screening, particularly in developing countries. The molecular mechanisms mediating the effect of the environment on CRC pathogenesis provide a new platform for the development of novel targets for screening. Animal experiments and larger studies in humans are still needed to elucidate the interplay of microbiota, the innate immune system, genetic factors, diet, and CRC before active intervention through the manipulation of gut microbiota can occur. Noninvasive blood tests, such as the measure of plasmic methylated septin-9, have potential as screening tools for CRC, due to the possibility of improving population compliance to CRC screening compared to the collection of stool samples but insufficient performance remains a concern. The high population risk of CRC worldwide ensures the need for continued development in this area to reduce the associated morbidity and mortality.

References

Ahlquist DA, Skoletsky JE, Boynton KA, et al. Colorectal cancer screening by detection of altered human DNA in stool: feasibility of a multitarget assay panel. Gastroenterology. 2000;119:1219–27.

Ahn J, Sinha R, Pei Z, et al. Human gut microbiome and risk for colorectal cancer. J Natl Cancer Inst. 2013;105:1907–11.

Allison JE, Tekawa IS, Ransom LJ, et al. A comparison of fecal occult-blood tests for colorectal-cancer screening. N Engl J Med. 1996;334:155–9.

Benard F, Barkun AN, Martel M, et al. Systematic review of colorectal cancer screening guidelines for average-risk adults: summarizing the current global recommendations. World J Gastroenterol. 2018;24:124–38.

Bishehsari F, Mahdavinia M, Vacca M, et al. Epidemiological transition of colorectal cancer in developing countries: environmental factors, molecular pathways, and opportunities for prevention. World J Gastroenterol. 2014;20:6055–72.

Brenner H, Stock C, Hoffmeister M. Effect of screening sigmoidoscopy and screening colonoscopy on colorectal cancer incidence and mortality: systematic review and meta-analysis of randomised controlled trials and observational studies. BMJ. 2014;348:g2467.

Carroll MR, Seaman HE, Halloran SP. Tests and investigations for colorectal cancer screening. Clin Biochem. 2014;47:921–39.

Chen LS, Yen AM, Chiu SY, et al. Baseline faecal occult blood concentration as a predictor of incident colorectal neoplasia: longitudinal follow-up of a Taiwanese population-based colorectal cancer screening cohort. Lancet Oncol. 2011;12:551–8.

Chiang TH, Lee YC, Tu CH, et al. Performance of the immunochemical fecal occult blood test in predicting lesions in the lower gastrointestinal tract. CMAJ. 2011;183:1474–81.

Chiang TH, Chuang SL, Chen SL, et al. Difference in performance of fecal immunochemical tests with the same hemoglobin cutoff concentration in a nationwide colorectal cancer screening program. Gastroenterology. 2014;147:1317–26.

Chiu HM, Lee YC, Tu CH, et al. Association between early stage colon neoplasms and false-negative results from the fecal immunochemical test. Clin Gastroenterol Hepatol. 2013;11:832–8 e1-2.

Chiu HM, Chen SL, Yen AM, et al. Effectiveness of fecal immunochemical testing in reducing colorectal cancer mortality from the one million Taiwanese screening program. Cancer. 2015;121:3221–9.

Chiu HM, Ching JY, Wu KC, et al. A risk-scoring system combined with a fecal immunochemical test is effective in screening high-risk subjects for early colonoscopy to detect advanced colorectal neoplasms. Gastroenterology. 2016;150:617–25 e3.

Church TR, Wandell M, Lofton-Day C, et al. Prospective evaluation of methylated SEPT9 in plasma for detection of asymptomatic colorectal cancer. Gut. 2014;63:317–25.

Eliakim R, Yassin K, Niv Y, et al. Prospective multicenter performance evaluation of the second-generation colon capsule compared with colonoscopy. Endoscopy. 2009;41:1026–31.

Elshimali YI, Khaddour H, Sarkissyan M, et al. The clinical utilization of circulating cell free DNA (CCFDNA) in blood of cancer patients. Int J Mol Sci. 2013;14:18925–58.

Gagniere J, Raisch J, Veziant J, et al. Gut microbiota imbalance and colorectal cancer. World J Gastroenterol. 2016;22:501–18.

Gezer U, Yoruker EE, Keskin M, et al. Histone methylation marks on circulating nucleosomes as novel blood-based biomarker in colorectal cancer. Int J Mol Sci. 2015;16:29654–62.

Grobbee EJ, van der Vlugt M, van Vuuren AJ, et al. A randomised comparison of two faecal immunochemical tests in population-based colorectal cancer screening. Gut. 2017;66:1975–82.

Hassan C, Giorgi Rossi P, Camilloni L, et al. Meta-analysis: adherence to colorectal cancer screening and the detection rate for advanced neoplasia, according to the type of screening test. Aliment Pharmacol Ther. 2012;36:929–40.

Hundt S, Haug U, Brenner H. Comparative evaluation of immunochemical fecal occult blood tests for colorectal adenoma detection. Ann Intern Med. 2009;150:162–9.

Imperiale TF, Ransohoff DF, Itzkowitz SH, et al. Multitarget stool DNA testing for colorectal-cancer screening. N Engl J Med. 2014;370:1287–97.

Inadomi JM, Vijan S, Janz NK, et al. Adherence to colorectal cancer screening: a randomized clinical trial of competing strategies. Arch Intern Med. 2012;172:575–82.

Inra JA, Syngal S. Colorectal cancer in young adults. Dig Dis Sci. 2015;60:722–33.

Johnson CD, Chen MH, Toledano AY, et al. Accuracy of CT colonography for detection of large adenomas and cancers. N Engl J Med. 2008;359:1207–17.

Kay CL, Evangelou HA. A review of the technical and clinical aspects of virtual endoscopy. Endoscopy. 1996;28:768–75.

Khalid-de Bakker CA, Jonkers DM, Sanduleanu S, et al. Test performance of immunologic fecal occult blood testing and sigmoidoscopy compared with primary colonoscopy screening for colorectal advanced adenomas. Cancer Prev Res (Phila). 2011;4:1563–71.

Knudsen AB, Zauber AG, Rutter CM, et al. Estimation of benefits, burden, and harms of colorectal cancer screening strategies: modeling study for the US preventive services task force. JAMA. 2016;315:2595–609.

Lee JK, Liles EG, Bent S, et al. Accuracy of fecal immunochemical tests for colorectal cancer: systematic review and meta-analysis. Ann Intern Med. 2014;160:171.

Lee YC, Li-Sheng Chen S, Ming-Fang Yen A, et al. Association between colorectal cancer mortality and gradient fecal hemoglobin concentration in colonoscopy noncompliers. J Natl Cancer Inst 2017;109.

Lee YC, Hsu CY, Chen SL, et al. Effects of screening and universal healthcare on long-term colorectal cancer mortality. Int J Epidemiol. 2019a;48:538–48.

Lee YC, Fann JC, Chiang TH, et al. Time to colonoscopy and risk of colorectal cancer in patients with positive results from fecal immunochemical tests. Clin Gastroenterol Hepatol. 2019b;17:1332–40.

Locker GY, Hamilton S, Harris J, et al. ASCO 2006 update of recommendations for the use of tumor markers in gastrointestinal cancer. J Clin Oncol. 2006;24:5313–27.

Lofton-Day C, Model F, Devos T, et al. DNA methylation biomarkers for blood-based colorectal cancer screening. Clin Chem. 2008;54:414–23.

Niedermaier T, Weigl K, Hoffmeister M, et al. Flexible sigmoidoscopy in colorectal cancer screening: implications of different colonoscopy referral strategies. Eur J Epidemiol. 2018;33:473–84.

Nishihara R, Wu K, Lochhead P, et al. Long-term colorectal-cancer incidence and mortality after lower endoscopy. N Engl J Med. 2013;369:1095–105.

Pickhardt PJ. Incidence of colonic perforation at CT colonography: review of existing data and implications for screening of asymptomatic adults. Radiology. 2006;239:313–6.

Rex DK, Lieberman DA. Feasibility of colonoscopy screening: discussion of issues and recommendations regarding implementation. Gastrointest Endosc. 2001;54:662–7.

Rex DK, Adler SN, Aisenberg J, et al. Accuracy of capsule colonoscopy in detecting colorectal polyps in a screening population. Gastroenterology. 2015;148:948–57 e2.

Rex DK, Boland CR, Dominitz JA, et al. Colorectal cancer screening: recommendations for physicians and patients from the U.S. multi-society task force on colorectal cancer. Gastroenterology. 2017;153:307–23.

Rockey DC. Occult gastrointestinal bleeding. N Engl J Med. 1999;341:38–46.

Rockey DC, Paulson E, Niedzwiecki D, et al. Analysis of air contrast barium enema, computed tomographic colonography, and colonoscopy: prospective comparison. Lancet. 2005;365:305–11.

Siegel RL, Miller KD, Fedewa SA, et al. Colorectal cancer statistics, 2017. CA Cancer J Clin. 2017;67:177–93.

Song L, Jia J, Peng X, et al. The performance of the SEPT9 gene methylation assay and a comparison with other CRC screening tests: a meta-analysis. Sci Rep. 2017;7:3032.

Stoop EM, de Haan MC, de Wijkerslooth TR, et al. Participation and yield of colonoscopy versus non-cathartic CT colonography in population-based screening for colorectal cancer: a randomised controlled trial. Lancet Oncol. 2012;13:55–64.

Sung JJ, Lau JY, Young GP, et al. Asia Pacific consensus recommendations for colorectal cancer screening. Gut. 2008;57:1166–76.

Tinmouth J, Lansdorp-Vogelaar I, Allison JE. Faecal immunochemical tests versus guaiac faecal occult blood tests: what clinicians and colorectal cancer screening programme organisers need to know. Gut. 2015;64:1327–37.

Van Gossum A, Munoz-Navas M, Fernandez-Urien I, et al. Capsule endoscopy versus colonoscopy for the detection of polyps and cancer. N Engl J Med. 2009;361:264–70.

Wong MC, John GK, Hirai HW, et al. Changes in the choice of colorectal cancer screening tests in primary care settings from 7,845 prospectively collected surveys. Cancer Causes Control. 2012;23:1541–8.

Wong MC, Ching JY, Chan VC, et al. Informed choice vs. no choice in colorectal cancer screening tests: a prospective cohort study in real-life screening practice. Am J Gastroenterol. 2014;109:1072–9.

Wong SH, Kwong TNY, Chow TC, et al. Quantitation of faecal *Fusobacterium* improves faecal immunochemical test in detecting advanced colorectal neoplasia. Gut. 2017;66:1441–8.

Zauber AG, Winawer SJ, O'Brien MJ, et al. Colonoscopic polypectomy and long-term prevention of colorectal-cancer deaths. N Engl J Med. 2012;366:687–96.

Zhu MM, Xu XT, Nie F, et al. Comparison of immunochemical and guaiac-based fecal occult blood test in screening and surveillance for advanced colorectal neoplasms: a meta-analysis. J Dig Dis. 2010;11:148–60.

Endoscopy-Based Colorectal Cancer Screening

Masau Sekiguchi and Takahisa Matsuda

Abstract

Screening sigmoidoscopy has been shown to reduce colorectal cancer (CRC) mortality and incidence in several randomized controlled trials (RCTs). However, its effect on the proximal colon is limited, and screening colonoscopy is expected to be more effective for this region. Despite the lack of evidence from RCTs, a reduction in CRC mortality and incidence by screening colonoscopy has been demonstrated in high-quality case-control and cohort studies, while several RCTs examining the effectiveness of screening colonoscopy are ongoing. Both sigmoidoscopy and colonoscopy are reportedly safe; however, continuous monitoring should be undertaken particularly for screening colonoscopy because of its invasiveness. With accumulating evidence on its effectiveness and safety, increased implementation of colonoscopy-based CRC screening is predicted. To maximize the effectiveness of this screening approach, achieving high detectability of colonoscopy is essential. In this sense, methods to increase the detectability of colonoscopy, such as add-on devices and image-enhanced endoscopy as well as good bowel cleansing, should be elucidated.

Keywords

Bowel cleansing · Colonoscopy · Colorectal cancer · Image-enhanced endoscopy Mortality reduction · Perforation Sigmoidoscopy

4.1 Introduction

In colorectal cancer (CRC) screening, it is essential to utilize colonoscopy efficiently because of its advantages in visualizing colorectal lesions directly and enabling simultaneous polypectomy for detected colorectal polyps. However, colonoscopy is a relatively invasive procedure and its capacity as examination resource is limited. Therefore, the approach by which to implement colonoscopy in colorectal cancer screening should be carefully considered, with sufficient regard to its effectiveness, safety, resource capacity, and cost-effectiveness.

Currently, with the development and widespread use of colonoscopy in clinical practice, increasing attention is being focused on

M. Sekiguchi (✉) · T. Matsuda
Cancer Screening Center, National Cancer Center Hospital, Tokyo, Japan

Endoscopy Division, National Cancer Center Hospital, Tokyo, Japan

Division of Screening Technology, Center for Public Health Sciences, National Cancer Center, Tokyo, Japan

© Springer Nature Singapore Pte Ltd. 2021
H.-M. Chiu, H.-H. Chen (eds.), *Colorectal Cancer Screening*,
https://doi.org/10.1007/978-981-15-7482-5_4

colonoscopy-based screening in which colonoscopy is used as the primary screening tool, in addition to CRC screening using noninvasive tests such as the guaiac fecal occult blood test (gFOBT) and the fecal immunochemical test (FIT). In this chapter, evidence on the effectiveness and safety of colonoscopy-based screening, the current situation and future perspectives of colonoscopy-based screening conducted globally, and methods to increase the effectiveness of screening colonoscopy are reviewed.

4.2   Effectiveness of Lower Endoscopy Screening

4.2.1   Colonoscopy

Among several measurements of CRC screening effectiveness, the reduction in CRC mortality is the most direct and important. Test performance measurements of screening modalities, such as sensitivity and specificity for CRC and colorectal neoplasia, should also be understood. The screening sensitivity of a single-session total colonoscopy is known to be very high; the sensitivity for advanced colorectal neoplasia (ACN) is reportedly 88%–98% and that for CRC is 92%–99%, higher than any other screening test (Zauber et al. 2008; Lieberman 2009; Schreuders et al. 2015). Because of this high detectability, there has been a great expectation for the reduction in CRC mortality by screening colonoscopy.

Despite the lack of evidence from randomized controlled trials (RCTs), extensive evidence of the CRC mortality reduction effect of colonoscopy have been accumulated from high-quality cohort studies and case-control studies, as shown in Table 4.1 (Baxter et al. 2009; Kahi et al. 2009; Manser et al. 2012; Nishihara et al. 2013; Doubeni et al. 2018). The reduction in CRC incidence also has been reported from several cohort and case-control studies (Table 4.2) (Kahi et al. 2009; Manser et al. 2012; Nishihara et al. 2013; Cotterchio et al. 2005; Brenner et al. 2010; Doubeni et al. 2013; Brenner et al. 2014). This effect is believed to be largely attributable to the endoscopic removal of colorectal neoplastic lesions. The effect of polypectomy on CRC incidence and mortality has been well examined and demonstrated in several case-control and cohort studies, including the National Polyp Study (NPS) (Brenner et al. 2011; Winawer et al. 1993; Zauber et al. 2012). The NPS was a US multicenter postpolypectomy surveillance study of patients with one or more adenomas. From the NPS, in 1993 Winawer et al. reported the effect of polypectomy on reducing CRC incidence by evaluating CRC incidence in 1418 patients who had undergone a complete colonoscopy in which all adenomas were removed endoscopically and comparing it with the incidence of three reference groups (two cohorts with no resected colorectal polyps and one general population registry) (Winawer et al. 1993). As a result, a reduction in CRC incidence of 76%–90% was indicated. Zauber et al. also recently reported the CRC mortality-reducing effect of polypectomy by analyzing the CRC mortality data of the NPS cohort (Zauber et al. 2012). The mortality was compared with the expected incidence-based CRC mortality in a reference group estimated from the database of the Surveillance, Epidemiology, and End Results (SEER) program. As compared with the reference group, a CRC mortality reduction of 53% was observed in the adenoma cohort after a median follow-up of 15.8 years. Furthermore, the study showed that CRC mortality was similar between the adenoma cohort and the non-adenoma cohort during 10 years of follow-up after polypectomy, indicating that the effectiveness of polypectomy may last for 10 years.

Among the studies shown in Table 4.1, the large prospective, observational cohort study by Nishihara et al. has provided the strongest evidence on the effectiveness of screening colonoscopy (Nishihara et al. 2013). They assessed the association between the use of lower endoscopy (sigmoidoscopy and colonoscopy) and CRC mortality and incidence using the data from two large cohorts (the Nurses' Health Study and the Health Professional Follow-up study). As shown in Table 4.1, the study found that colonoscopy was associated with a CRC mortality reduction of 68% (adjusted hazard ratio (aHR) 0.32; 95% con-

Table 4.1 Evidence on CRC mortality reduction by screening colonoscopy

References	Authors	Report year	Study design	HR or OR for CRC mortality (95% CI)		
				Whole colon	Distal colon	Proximal colon
Baxter et al. (2009)	Baxter et al.	2009	Case-control study	0.69 (0.63–0.74)	0.33 (0.28–0.39)	0.99 (0.86–1.14)
Kahi et al. (2009)	Kahi et al.	2009	Cohort study	0.35 (0–1.06)	–	–
Manser et al. (2012)	Manser et al.	2012	Cohort study	0.12 (0.01–0.93)	–	–
Nishihara et al. (2013)	Nishihara et al.	2013	Cohort study	0.32 (0.24–0.45)	0.18 (0.10–0.31)	0.47 (0.29–0.76)
Doubeni et al. (2018)	Doubeni et al.	2018	Case-control study	0.33 (0.21–0.52)	0.25 (0.12–0.53)	0.35 (0.18–0.65)

CI confidence interval, *CRC* colorectal cancer, *HR* hazard ratio, *OR* odds ratio

Table 4.2 Evidence on CRC incidence reduction by screening colonoscopy

References	Authors	Report year	Study design	HR or OR for CRC incidence (95% CI)		
				Whole colon	Distal colon	Proximal colon
Cotterchio et al. (2005)	Cotterchio et al.	2005	Case-control study	0.69 (0.44–1.07)	0.68 (0.49–0.99)	1.02 (0.72–1.45)
Kahi et al. (2009)	Kahi et al.	2009	Cohort study	0.52 (0.22–0.82)	–	–
Brenner et al. (2010)	Brenner et al.	2010	Cohort study	0.52 (0.37–0.73)	0.33 (0.21–0.53)	1.05 (0.63–1.76)
Manser et al. (2012)	Manser et al.	2012	Cohort study	0.31 (0.16–0.57)	–	–
Nishihara et al. (2013)	Nishihara et al.	2013	Cohort study (negative colonoscopy)	0.44 (0.38–0.52)	0.24 (0.18–0.32)	0.73 (0.57–0.92)
			(Polypctomy)	0.57 (0.45–0.72)	0.40 (0.27–0.59)	0.83 (0.59–1.18)
Doubeni et al. (2013)	Doubeni et al.[a]	2013	Case-control study	0.29 (0.15–0.58)	0.26 (0.06–1.11)	0.36 (0.16–0.80)
Brenner et al. (2014)	Brenner et al.	2014	Case-control study	0.09 (0.07–0.13)	0.05 (0.03–0.08)	0.22 (0.14–0.33)

CI confidence interval, *CRC* colorectal cancer, *HR* hazard ratio, *OR* odds ratio
[a]The incidence of late-stage CRC was evaluated

fidence interval (CI) 0.24–0.45) as compared with no lower endoscopy. The effect of colonoscopy on reducing CRC mortality seems stronger in the distal colon; in the proximal and distal colon, CRC mortality following colonoscopy was reduced by 53% (aHR 0.47; 95% CI 0.29–0.76) and 82% (aHR 0.18; 95% CI 0.10–0.31), respectively. The study also showed the association between colonoscopy and CRC incidence reduction as compared with no lower endoscopy. Although negative colonoscopy not requiring polypectomy was significantly related with CRC incidence reduction in both the proximal (aHR 0.73; 95% CI: 0.57–0.92) and distal colon (aHR 0.24; 95% CI: 0.18–0.32), a significant relationship between colonoscopy with polypectomy and reduced CRC incidence was only observed in the distal colon (aHR 0.40; 95% CI: 0.27–0.59) and not in the proximal colon (aHR 0.83; 95% CI: 0.59–1.18). The discrepancy in the effect from colonoscopy between the proximal and distal colon was indicated, as observed in several other studies (Baxter et al. 2009; Nishihara et al. 2013; Cotterchio et al. 2005; Brenner et al. 2010). Several factors may be involved in this discrepancy, such as the quality of colonoscopy and polypectomy and differences in the CRC biological characteristics according to location. Further research is required on this issue, and in this sense, the results from subsequent RCTs are warranted.

Currently, several large-scale RCTs evaluating the effect of screening colonoscopy on CRC mortality are ongoing, as shown in Table 4.3. Trials in Spain (COLONPREV) (Quintero et al. 2012) and the United States (the Colonoscopy vs. Fecal immunochemical Test in Reducing Mortality from Colorectal Cancer: CONFIRM) (U.S. Department of Veterans Affairs) are comparing one-time screening colonoscopy with the fecal immunochemical test (FIT). Uniquely, a Japanese trial (Akita pop-colon trial) (Saito et al. 2020) is investigating one-time screening colonoscopy followed by annual FIT. In addition, two trials are comparing screening colonoscopy with no screening. A European trial (the Nordic-European Initiative on Colorectal Cancer: NordICC) (Kaminski et al. 2012) is examining the benefit of one-time screening colonoscopy

Table 4.3 Ongoing RCTs on the effectiveness of screening colonoscopy

	Study	Country	Target age	Study design	Starting year	Scheduled observation period
Quintero et al. (2012)	COLONPREV	Spain	50–69 years	RCT	2008	10 years
				Intervention arm: One-round CS		
				Control arm: FIT (biannual)		
Saito et al. (2020)	Akita pop-colon trial	Japan	40–74 years	RCT	2009	10 years
				Intervention arm:One-round CS + FIT (annual)		
				Control arm: FIT (annual)		
Kaminski et al. (2012)	NordICC	The Netherlands, Norway, Poland, etc.	55–64 years	RCT	2009	10–15 years
				Intervention arm: One-round CS		
				Control arm: No screening		
	CONFIRM	United States	50–75 years	RCT	2012	10 years
				Intervention arm: One-round CS		
				Control arm:FIT (annual)		
	SCREESCO	Sweden	59–62 years	RCT	2014	15 years
				Intervention arm 1: One-round CS		
				Intervention arm 2: FIT (years 1 and 3)		
				Control arm: No screening		

CS colonoscopy, *FIT* fecal immunochemical test, *RCT* randomized controlled trial

compared with no screening, while a Swedish trial (Screening of Swedish Colons: SCREESCO) (Uppsala University Hospital) has three arms comprising screening colonoscopy, FIT, and no screening. The results of these RCTs are expected to be available between 2020 and 2030 to provide conclusive findings on the effectiveness of screening colonoscopy.

4.2.2 Flexible Sigmoidoscopy

The positive effect of screening sigmoidoscopy on CRC mortality and incidence was clearly proved by four RCTs (Table 4.4) (Atkin et al. 2010, 2017; Segnan et al. 2011; Schoen et al. 2012; Holme et al. 2014). As shown in Table 4.4, in three RCTs, a UK trial (UKSST), a US trial (PLCO), and a Norwegian trial (NORCCAP), overall CRC mor-

Table 4.4 Evidence on CRC mortality and incidence reduction by screening sigmoidoscopy in RCTs

Study	Country	Target age	Study design	No. of participants	Observed period	HR for CRC mortality (95%CI)	HR for CRC incidence (95%CI)
UFKSST	UK	55–64 years	RCT		17.1 years	Whole colon 0.70 (0.62–0.79)	Whole colon 0.74 (0.70–0.80)
			Intervention group: one-round SIG	57,099		Distal colon 0.54 (0.45–0.65)	Distal colon 0.59 (0.54–0.64)
			Control group: no screening	112,939		Proximal colon 0.91 (0.76–1.08)	Proximal colon 0.96 (0.87–1.06)
SCORE	Italy	5–64 years	RCT		11.4 years	Whole colon 0.78 (0.56–1.08)	Whole colon 0.82 (0.69–0.96)
			Intervention group: one-round SIG	17,136		Distal colon 0.73 (0.47–1.12)	Distal colon 0.76 (0.62–0.94)
			Control group: no screening	17,144		Proximal colon 0.85 (0.52–1.39)	Proximal colon 0.91 (0.69–1.20)
PLCO	USA	55–74 years	RCT		11.9 years	Whole colon 0.74 (0.63–0.87)	Whole colon 0.79 (0.72–0.85)
			Intervention group: two-rounds SIG	77,445		Distal colon 0.50 (0.38–0.64)	Distal colon 0.71 (0.64–0.80)
			Control group: no screening	77,455		Proximal colon 0.97 (0.77–1.22)	Proximal colon 0.86 (0.76–0.97)
NORCCAP	Norway	50–64 years	RCT		10.9 years	Whole colon 0.73 (0.56–0.94)	Whole colon 0.80 (0.70–0.92)
			Intervention group: one-round SIG (without/with FIT)	20,572		Distal colon 0.79 (0.55–1.11)	Distal colon 0.76 (0.63–0.92)
			Control group: no screening	78,220		Proximal colon 0.73 (0.49–1.09)	Proximal colon 0.90 (0.73–1.10)

CI confidence interval, *CRC* colorectal cancer, *FIT* fecal immunochemical test, *HR* hazard ratio, *RCT* randomized controlled trial, *SIG* sigmoidoscopy

tality was significantly reduced by approximately 30% by screening sigmoidoscopy. Even in an Italian trial (SCORE) in which the statistically significant effect of overall CRC mortality reduction was not proven in the intention-to-treat analysis, significant CRC mortality reduction was demonstrated in the per-protocol analysis (HR 0.69, 95%CI: 0.40–0.96) (Segnan et al. 2011). In all four RCTs, a statistically significant reduction in overall CRC incidence of approximately 20% was clearly demonstrated.

In these four RCTs, the adherence to sigmoidoscopy was high (around 60%–80%), the number of screening sigmoidoscopy sessions was one or two, and the observation period was over 10 years. With consideration of these facts, it can be postulated that the effect of screening sigmoidoscopy lasts more than 10 years.

Differences in the effects on CRC mortality and incidence according to location (proximal and distal colon) were evaluated in all four RCTs. It was clearly shown that the main effect of sigmoidoscopy was in the distal colon, as can be easily imagined from the nature of the procedure. However, a significant reduction in CRC mortality and incidence by sigmoidoscopy in the proximal colon was not clarified from these RCTs. Although sigmoidoscopy is an effective screening procedure with high-level evidence from RCTs, its limitations in terms of its insufficient effectiveness in the proximal colon should be understood.

4.3   Safety of Screening Lower Endoscopy

4.3.1   Colonoscopy

Particularly in screening, safety assurances are essential because the target population of screening is healthy individuals. Therefore, noninvasive and safe screening tests are preferred in the screening setting. Thus, careful attention should be paid to screening colonoscopy because it is a relatively invasive procedure compared with other non-invasive tests such as gFOBT and FIT.

Bleeding and perforation are two major complications known to be related to colonoscopy. A systematic review and meta-analysis of population-based studies examining post-colonoscopy examinations (within 30 days after the procedure) showed that the frequencies of bleeding, perforation, and mortality were 2.6 per 1000 (95% CI 1.7–3.7), 0.5 per 1000 (95% CI 0.4–0.7), and 2.9 per 100,000 (95% CI 1.1–5.5) colonoscopies, respectively (Reumkens et al. 2016). Polypectomy is more associated with these complications than observational colonoscopy alone, and the meta-analysis found that the frequencies of post-polypectomy bleeding and perforation were 9.8 per 1000 (95% CI 7.7–12.1) and 0.8 per 1000 (95% CI 0.6–1.0), respectively, which were higher than those of observational colonoscopy. The frequencies of bleeding and perforation of colonoscopy without polypectomy were reportedly 0.6 per 1000 (95% CI 0.2–1.1) and 0.4 per 1000 (95% CI 0.2–0.8), respectively. Regarding these major complications, several worldwide societies of gastrointestinal endoscopy and gastroenterology have set performance targets for colonoscopy safety. For example, the American Society for Gastrointestinal Endoscopy (ASGE) and the American College of Gastroenterology (ACG) Task Force on Quality in Endoscopy have stated that post-colonoscopy perforation should be ≤1/500 colonoscopies (all examinations) and ≤1/1000 (screening examinations), and that post-polypectomy bleeding should be ≤1/100 colonoscopies (Rex et al. 2015). The reported prevalence from the abovementioned meta-analysis was lower than these standards, suggesting that colonoscopy is a safe procedure. However, considering that mortality is still observed, albeit at a low frequency, and that reported complication frequencies from clinical trials tend to be lower than those in real clinical practice settings due to many physicians with variable technique levels conducting colonoscopic procedures, continuous careful attention is required for the safety of colonoscopy.

Recently, with the increasing number of high-risk individuals undergoing screening for CRC, such as the elderly, those with comorbidities, and those taking antithrombotic drugs, a potentially increased risk of non-gastrointestinal complications following colonoscopy, such as cardiovascular, pulmonary, and neurovascular events, has been reported (Johnson et al. 2017). It is extremely important to carefully consider whether colonoscopy should be performed in such high-risk individuals by balancing the benefits and risks of the procedure. Despite this situation, however, it is not believed that the risk of non-gastrointestinal complications is a compelling reason for opposing the use of colonoscopy for screening. A recent large-scale population-based study in the United States reported that the rates of severe non-gastrointestinal complications following colonoscopy are sufficiently low (Wang et al. 2018).

4.3.2 Flexible Sigmoidoscopy

Flexible sigmoidoscopy is a less invasive procedure than colonoscopy, requiring more limited bowel preparation and no sedation. A meta-analysis reported a low risk of bleeding and perforation resulting from screening sigmoidoscopy (Lin et al. 2016). The frequencies of bleeding and perforation of screening sigmoidoscopy were found to be 0.2 per 1000 (95% CI 0.07–0.4) and 0.1 per 1000 (95% CI 0.04–0.14), respectively. However, screening sigmoidoscopy requires follow-up diagnostic colonoscopy for individuals with positive findings, and if the complication frequencies are calculated with follow-up colonoscopy, the frequencies increase. A meta-analysis showed that the pooled prevalence of bleeding and perforation of the follow-up colonoscopy was 3.4 per 1000 (95% CI 0.5–6.3) and 1.4 per 1000 (95% CI 0.9–2.6), respectively (Lin et al. 2016).

4.4 Current Situation and Future Perspectives on the Global Implementation of Screening Colonoscopy

In many countries, total colonoscopy is mainly used as a follow-up diagnostic test for individuals with positive results from noninvasive screening tests (Schreuders et al. 2015). For instance, in Japan, Taiwan, and many other countries, FIT is used as a primary screening tool in population-based screening, and colonoscopy is performed for those with a positive FIT (Table 4.5).

However, in addition to the use of colonoscopy as a follow-up test, with the collective evidence on its effectiveness and safety, colonoscopy has been increasingly adopted as a primary screening tool for CRC, as shown in Table 4.5 (Schreuders et al. 2015). In countries, such as the United States and Germany, where colonoscopy has been widely used as a primary screening tool, declining CRC mortality and incidence have been observed (Chen et al. 2018). However, an important point regarding screening colonoscopy is the relatively lower acceptability among screening populations than other noninvasive screening tests. From the experience in Germany, the annual participation rate for CRC screening with colonoscopy was reportedly only around 2% and the calculated cumulative participation rate over the first 6 years was only around 13% (Pox et al. 2012).

Considering the limited examination resource of colonoscopies and low preference among screening individuals, the selection of individuals at high risk for colorectal neoplasia and requiring colonoscopy is believed to be helpful for the more efficient future use of screening colonoscopy. Scoring systems to predict advanced colorectal neoplasia, including the Asia Pacific Colorectal Screening Score (Table 4.6), have been reported to be useful for the selection of high-risk individuals (Yeoh et al. 2011; Kaminski et al. 2014a; Wong et al. 2016; Sung et al. 2018; Sekiguchi et al. 2018; Peng et al. 2018). In addition, the combined use of FIT and such scores may enable more efficient CRC screening (Chiu et al. 2016). With these useful items, more efficient utilization of screening colonoscopy for CRC screening is expected.

4.5 Methods to Increase Effectiveness of Screening Colonoscopy

It is essential to detect colorectal neoplasia correctly to maximize the effectiveness of colonoscopy. In fact, the adenoma detection rate (ADR),

Table 4.5 Current situation of colonoscopy-based CRC screening worldwide (Schreuders et al. 2015)

Country	Target regions	Program type	Starting year	Target age (years)	Screening interval (months)	Other screening options
European region						
Austria	All	Opportunistic	2005	50+	84–120	gFOBT
Czech Republic	All	Opportunistic	2010	55+	120	FIT
Germany	All	Opportunistic	2002	55+	120	gFOBT
Greece	All	Opportunistic		50–80		gFOBT
Luxembourg	All	Opportunistic	2005	50+		gFOBT
Norway	Regions	Organized	2012	50–64		FIT, SIG
Poland	All	Organized	2000	50–66	120	gFOBT
Slovakia	All	Opportunistic				gFOBT
Sweden	Regions	Organized				gFOBT, FIT
Switzerland	All	Opportunistic		50+		gFOBT
Turkey	All	Opportunistic	2009	50–74	120	FIT
Region of the Americas						
Argentina	Urban areas	Organized		50–74		FIT
Bahamas		Opportunistic				gFOBT, FIT
Barbados		Opportunistic				gFOBT, FIT
Jamaica		Opportunistic				
Puerto Rico		Opportunistic		50–75		gFOBT, SIG
Trinidad/Tobago		Opportunistic				gFOBT, FIT
USA	Kaiser Permanente North Carolina	Organized		50–75	120	FIT
	Veterans health administration	Organized		51–75	120	gFOBT, SIG
Asia-Pacific and Eastern Mediterranean region						
Brunei		Opportunistic				
China	Hong Kong	Organized	2003	50+		gFOBT
	Shanghai and Hangzhou regions etc.	Organized	2008	40–74		gFOBT etc
Jordan		Opportunistic		50+		gFOBT, FIT

FIT fecal immunochemical test, *gFOBT* guaiac fecal occult blood test, *SIG* sigmoidoscopy

Table 4.6 Asia-Pacific colorectal screening score (Yeoh et al. 2011)

Scoring items		Points
Age (years)	<50	0
	50–69	2
	≥70	3
Sex	Female	0
	Male	1
CRC family history in a first-degree relative	Absent	0
	Present	2
Smoking	Never	0
	Current or past	1

which is a representative quality measurement of colonoscopy, is known to be associated with CRC mortality (Kaminski et al. 2010; Kaminski et al. 2017). In this section, approaches to improve detectability of colonoscopy are discussed in three major areas.

4.5.1 Add-on Devices

In recent years, high-definition white light endoscopy has become the standard approach and has led to an improvement in detectability. Add-on devices have been explored to further improve this detectability.

One potentially effective device is a ~~transparent~~ cap that can be attached to the tip of the colonoscope. Currently, not only a transparent cap but also a black cap are available (Fig. 4.1a). Even when a black cap is attached to the colonoscope, endoscopic images are not disturbed by the cap (Fig. 4.1b). Cap-assisted colonoscopy is believed to reduce the blind colonic surface by depressing the haustral folds (Matsuda et al. 2017). Several meta-analyses demonstrated a higher polyp detection rate of cap-assisted colonoscopy than standard colonoscopy (Ng et al. 2012; He et al. 2013; Westwood et al. 2012). However, no significant difference in ADR was found between cap-assisted colonoscopy and standard colonoscopy, and the effectiveness of a cap in terms of increasing ADR is still controversial.

In addition to a cap, other devices have also been developed recently, and Endocuff (Arc Medical Design, UK) has been shown to be particularly useful (Matsuda et al. 2017; Rex et al. 2018; Biecker et al. 2015; Floer et al. 2014). It consists of two rings of soft, flexible projections or branches, and can be attached to the tip of colonoscopes. The branches of Endocuff are used for flattering the colonic folds to improve the visibility of colonic surface, including that behind folds. Several previous RCTs demonstrated higher ADR in Endocuff-assisted colonoscopy than standard colonoscopy (Biecker et al. 2015; Floer et al. 2014).

4.5.2 Image-Enhanced Endoscopy

Image-enhanced endoscopy (IEE) includes conventional chromoendoscopy and virtual chromoendoscopy. Indigo carmine dye is most frequently used in conventional chromoendoscopy and is a contrast dye that enhances the mucosal surface but is not absorbed in the mucosal glands. A meta-analysis demonstrated the higher detectability of pancolonic chromoendoscopy using indigo carmine dye; however, a longer withdrawal time is required (Brown et al. 2016). Thus, it is difficult to adopt pancolonic chromoendoscopy as the routine procedure in CRC screening due to the required workload.

Instead of pancolonic chromoendoscopy, virtual chromoendoscopy, is a recent candidate procedure that can be routinely used in screening colonoscopy. Virtual chromoendoscopy includes several technologies, such as narrow-band imaging (NBI), iScan, flexible spectral imaging color enhancement, autofluorescence imaging, blue laser imaging, and linked-color imaging (Matsuda et al. 2017). The usefulness of virtual chromoendoscopy for the diagnosis and characterization of colorectal neoplasia is widely known. However, its utility for improving detectability in screening colonoscopy is still controversial and its use during the whole withdrawal period of colonoscopy has not become the stan-

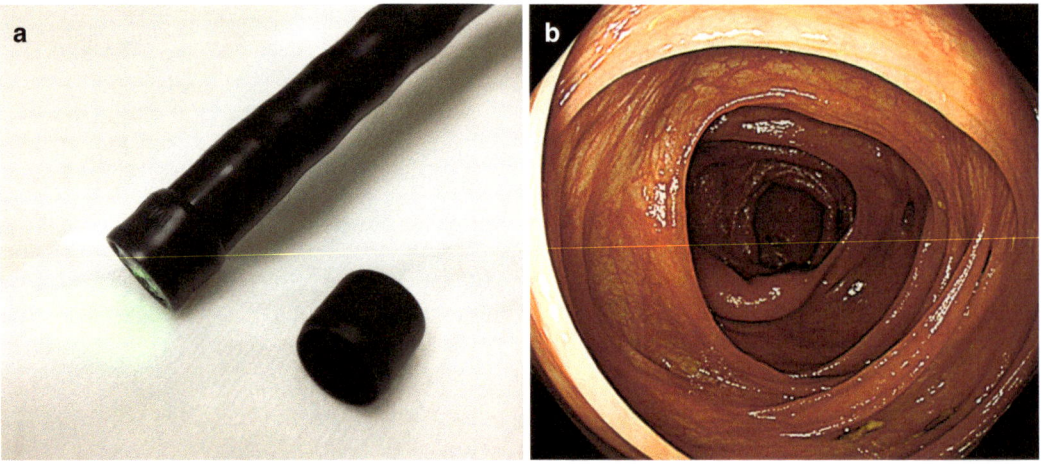

Fig. 4.1 Cap-assisted colonoscopy. (**a**) Black cap attached to the tip of a colonoscope. (**b**) Endoscopic image with a black cap attached to the tip of a colonoscope

dard method in screening colonoscopy. Although increasing studies reported the potential usefulness of virtual chromoendoscopy in terms of improving the detection of colorectal neoplasia, the pooled outcomes of the studies did not show the superiority of virtual chromoendoscopy over white-light imaging (Kaminski et al. 2014b; Omata et al. 2014; Nagorni et al. 2012). However, with the development of new technologies, this hurdle is expected to be overcome. Several years ago, second-generation NBI was developed with twofold brighter imaging, and a recent meta-analysis clearly demonstrated that it can yield a higher ADR than white-light imaging (Atkinson et al. 2019). Figure 4.2 shows the use of second-generation NBI in screening colonoscopy. A colon polyp can be easily detected as a well-demarcated brownish lesion using NBI, and the close view and combination use of the function of magnification are helpful for confirming the diagnosis.

4.5.3 Bowel Cleansing

Good bowel cleansing is an essential part of effective colonoscopy. If bowel preparation is inadequate, the detection and diagnosis of colorectal neoplasia are difficult, and important lesions including CRC may be missed.

Currently, several agents for colonoscopy preparation are available, as shown in Table 4.7 (Johnson et al. 2014; ASGE Standards of Practice Committee et al. 2015). High-volume polyethylene glycol (PEG) solutions have historically been the main agents, but low-volume agents have been developed and are now in wide use. A recent study comparing the real-world effectiveness of colonoscopy preparation agents found that MoviPrep, Suprep, and MiraLAX with Gatorade are associated with superior tolerability and bowel cleansing (Gu et al. 2019).

With regard to the timing of bowel preparation, there are two types: split-dose preparation and same-day preparation (Johnson et al. 2014; ASGE Standards of Practice Committee et al. 2015). In split-dose regimens, a proportion of the preparation agents are administered the day before and the remainder is administered on the day of colonoscopy, whereas, in same-day regimens, all preparation agents are administered in 1 day. Several previous meta-analyses demonstrated the favorable effect of split-dose regimens using high-volume PEG solutions, and such split-dose regimens have been recommended worldwide as being optimal (Johnson et al. 2014; ASGE Standards of Practice Committee et al. 2015; Martel et al. 2015; Enestvedt et al. 2012; Kilgore et al. 2011; Bucci et al. 2014). However, several studies have recently demonstrated no

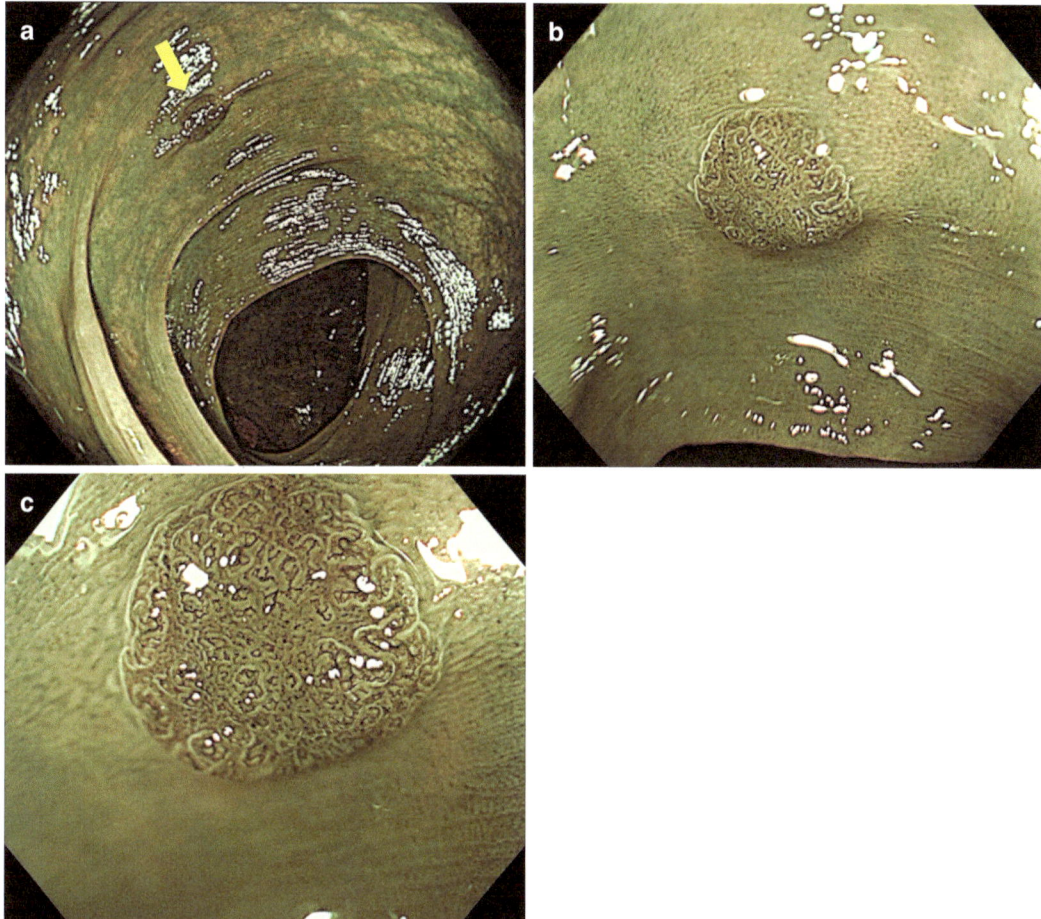

Fig. 4.2 Use of NBI in screening colonoscopy. (**a**) NBI image clearly visualizing a colon polyp is a well-demarcated brownish lesion. (**b**) Closer view using NBI. (**c**) Closer view with magnifying NBI: the lesion was confidently diagnosed as tubular adenoma, which is a good indication of polypectomy

Table 4.7 Bowel preparation agents

Bowel preparation agent	Composition	Regimen volume
PEG-ELS (GoLYTELY)	PEG, sodium sulfate, sodium, bicarbonate, sodium chloride, potassium chloride	4 L
Sulfate-free PEG-ELS (NuLYTELY)	PEG, sodium bicarbonate, sodium chloride, potassium chloride	4 L
Low-volume PEG-ELS with ascorbic acid (Moviprep)	PEG-3350, sodium sulfate, sodium chloride, ascorbic acid	2 L with 1 L clear liquid
Low-volume PEG-3350-SD (Miralax)	PEG-3350	238 g PEG-3350 with 2 L sports drink
Oral sodium sulfate (Suprep)	Sodium sulfate, potassium sulfate, magnesium sulfate	12 oz. with 2.5 L water
Magnesium citrate	Magnesium citrate	20–30 oz. with 2 L water
NaP tablets (Osmoprep)	Monobasic and dibasic NaP	32 tablets with 2 L water

inferiority in the effectiveness and better tolerance of same-day regimens (Cheng et al. 2018; Avalos et al. 2018). With regard to the preparation of same-day regimens, it is reportedly optimal to administer preparation agents on the day of colonoscopy than on the previous night (Chiu et al. 2006). Same-day regimens are now accepted as alternatives to split-dose regimens.

Evaluation and documentation of bowel preparation levels are also important. There are several evaluation scales, such as the Boston Bowel Preparation Scale, Ottawa Bowel Preparation Scale, and Aronchick Scale (ASGE Standards of Practice Committee et al. 2015). The first two scales are evaluated per colonic site and the last is evaluated for the whole colon.

Even with the development of preparation agents and regimens, inadequate bowel cleansing has been reported. However, there have also been reports of very favorable results for bowel preparation from several advanced institutions. For instance, good bowel preparation is reportedly achieved at the Cancer Screening Center of the National Cancer Center, Tokyo, Japan (Sekiguchi et al. 2019). In their recent paper, in which the data of screening colonoscopies at the Cancer Screening Center were used, approximately 99% of screened individuals scored 1–2 on the Aronchick Scale. A volume of 1800 ml of magnesium citrate or 2000 ml of polyethylene glycol was used on the day of colonoscopy. In addition, the administration of Moviprep has also recently been preferred on the day of colonoscopy. Their preparation method is very similar to the same-day method but given that sennoside (two tablets) is administered on the night before colonoscopy, the preparation method can be classified as a split-dose regimen in a wider sense. One reason for good bowel preparation can be explained by ethnicity, but there are also tips for good bowel preparation that can be applicable to other regions. One is that dedicated nurses are tasked to judge the adequacy of the bowel preparation before colonoscopy. If the bowel preparation is determined as inadequate by these nurses, additional preparation agents are administered. Another is that low-residue diets are used for 1–3 days before

colonoscopy for individuals with records of previous poor bowel preparation, previous abdominal surgery, or constipation.

4.6 Conclusions

In this chapter, the effectiveness and safety of screening lower endoscopy, the current situation and future perspectives on the global implementation of screening colonoscopy, and methods to increase the effectiveness of screening colonoscopy were reviewed. Accumulating evidence on the effectiveness and safety of screening colonoscopy indicates its future wide utilization. Efforts to increase detectability during procedures are strongly required to maximize the effectiveness of colonoscopy. Furthermore, sufficient consideration of factors other than effectiveness and safety, including acceptability among screening populations, cost-effectiveness, and limited capacity of endoscopic resources, is also essential for more efficient use of screening colonoscopy.

References

ASGE Standards of Practice Committee, Saltzman JR, Cash BD, Pasha SF, et al. Bowel preparation before colonoscopy. Gastrointest Endosc. 2015;81:781–94.

Atkin WS, Edwards R, Kralj-Hans I, et al. Once-only flexible sigmoidoscopy screening in prevention of colorectal cancer: a multicentre randomised controlled trial. Lancet. 2010;375:1624–33.

Atkin W, Wooldrage K, Parkin DM, et al. Long term effects of once-only flexible sigmoidoscopy screening after 17 years of follow-up: the UK flexible sigmoidoscopy screening randomised controlled trial. Lancet. 2017;389:1299–311.

Atkinson NSS, Ket S, Bassett P, et al. Narrow-band imaging for detection of neoplasia at colonoscopy: a meta-analysis of data from individual patients in randomized controlled trials. Gastroenterology. 2019;157:462–71.

Avalos DJ, Castro FJ, Zuckerman MJ, et al. Bowel preparations administered the morning of colonoscopy provide similar efficacy to a split dose regimen: a Meta analysis. J Clin Gastroenterol. 2018;52:859–68.

Baxter NN, Goldwasser MA, Paszat LF, et al. Association of colonoscopy and death from colorectal cancer. Ann Intern Med. 2009;150:1–8.

Biecker E, Floer M, Heinecke A, et al. Novel endocuff-assisted colonoscopy significantly increases the polyp detection rate: a randomized controlled trial. J Clin Gastroenterol. 2015;49:413–8.

Brenner H, Hoffmeister M, Arndt V, et al. Protection from right- and left-sided colorectal neoplasms after colonoscopy: population-based study. J Natl Cancer Inst. 2010;102:89–95.

Brenner H, Chang-Claude J, Seiler CM, et al. Protection from colorectal cancer after colonoscopy: a population-based, case-control study. Ann Intern Med. 2011;154:22–30.

Brenner H, Chang-Claude J, Jansen L, et al. Reduced risk of colorectal cancer up to 10 years after screening, surveillance, or diagnostic colonoscopy. Gastroenterology. 2014;146:709–17.

Brown SR, Baraza W, Din S, et al. Chromoscopy versus conventional endoscopy for the detection of polyps in the colon and rectum. Cochrane Database Syst Rev. 2016;4:CD006439.

Bucci C, Rotondano G, Hassan C, et al. Optimal bowel cleansing for colonoscopy: split the dose! A series of meta-analyses of controlled studies. Gastrointest Endosc. 2014;80:566–76.

Chen C, Stock C, Hoffmeister M, et al. Public health impact of colonoscopy use on colorectal cancer mortality in Germany and the United States. Gastrointest Endosc. 2018;87:213–21.

Cheng YL, Huang KW, Liao WC, et al. Same-day versus split-dose bowel preparation before colonoscopy: a meta-analysis. J Clin Gastroenterol. 2018;52:392–400.

Chiu HM, Lin JT, Wang HP, et al. The impact of colon preparation timing on colonoscopic detection of colorectal neoplasms—a prospective endoscopist-blinded randomized trial. Am J Gastroenterol. 2006;101:2719–25.

Chiu HM, Ching JY, Wu KC, et al. A risk-scoring system combined with a fecal immunochemical test is effective in screening high-risk subjects for early colonoscopy to detect advanced colorectal neoplasms. Gastroenterology. 2016;150:617–25.

Cotterchio M, Manno M, Klar N, et al. Colorectal screening is associated with reduced colorectal cancer risk: a case-control study within the population-based Ontario familial colorectal cancer registry. Cancer Causes Control. 2005;16:865–75.

Doubeni CA, Weinmann S, Adams K, et al. Screening colonoscopy and risk for incident late-stage colorectal cancer diagnosis in average-risk adults: a nested case-control study. Ann Intern Med. 2013;158:312–20.

Doubeni CA, Corley DA, Quinn VP, et al. Effectiveness of screening colonoscopy in reducing the risk of death from right and left colon cancer: a large community-based study. Gut. 2018;67:291–8.

Enestvedt BK, Tofani C, Laine LA, et al. 4-Liter split-dose polyethylene glycol is superior to other bowel preparations, based on systematic review and meta-analysis. Clin Gastroenterol Hepatol. 2012;10:1225–31.

Floer M, Biecker E, Fitzlaff R, et al. Higher adenoma detection rates with endocuff-assisted colonoscopy – a randomized controlled multicenter trial. PLoS One. 2014;9:e114267.

Gu P, Lew D, Oh SJ, et al. Comparing the real-world effectiveness of competing colonoscopy preparations: results of a prospective trial. Am J Gastroenterol. 2019;114:305–14.

He Q, Li JD, An SL, et al. Cap-assisted colonoscopy versus conventional colonoscopy: systematic review and meta-analysis. Int J Color Dis. 2013;28:279–81.

Holme Ø, Løberg M, Kalager M, et al. Effect of flexible sigmoidoscopy screening on colorectal cancer incidence and mortality: a randomized clinical trial. JAMA. 2014;312:606–15.

Johnson DA, Barkun AN, Cohen LB, US Multi-Society Task Force on Colorectal Cancer, et al. Optimizing adequacy of bowel cleansing for colonoscopy: recommendations from the US multi-society task force on colorectal cancer. Gastroenterology. 2014;147:903–24.

Johnson DA, Lieberman D, Inadomi JM, et al. Increased post-procedural non-gastrointestinal adverse events after outpatient colonoscopy in high-risk patients. Clin Gastroenterol Hepatol. 2017;15:883–91.

Kahi CJ, Imperiale TF, Juliar BE, et al. Effect of screening colonoscopy on colorectal cancer incidence and mortality. Clin Gastroenterol Hepatol. 2009;7:770–5.

Kaminski MF, Regula J, Kraszewska E, et al. Quality indicators for colonoscopy and the risk of interval cancer. N Engl J Med. 2010;362:1795–803.

Kaminski MF, Bretthauer M, Zauber AG, et al. The NordICC study: rationale and design of a randomized trial on colonoscopy screening for colorectal cancer. Endoscopy. 2012;44:695–702.

Kaminski MF, Polkowski M, Kraszewska E, et al. A score to estimate the likelihood of detecting advanced colorectal neoplasia at colonoscopy. Gut. 2014a;63:1112–9.

Kaminski MF, Hassan C, Bisschops R, et al. Advanced imaging for detection and differentiation of colorectal neoplasia: European Society of Gastrointestinal Endoscopy (ESGE) guideline. Endoscopy. 2014b;46:435–49.

Kaminski MF, Wieszczy P, Rupinski M, et al. Increased rate of adenoma detection associates with reduced risk of colorectal cancer and death. Gastroenterology. 2017;153:98–105.

Kilgore TW, Abdinoor AA, Szary NM, et al. Bowel preparation with split-dose polyethylene glycol before colonoscopy: a meta-analysis of randomized controlled trials. Gastrointest Endosc. 2011;73:1240–5.

Lieberman DA. Clinical practice. Screening for colorectal cancer. N Engl J Med. 2009;361:1179–87.

Lin JS, Piper MA, Perdue LA, et al. Screening for colorectal cancer: updated evidence report and systematic review for the US preventive services task force. JAMA. 2016;315:2576–94.

Manser CN, Bachmann LM, Brunner J, et al. Colonoscopy screening and carcinoma-related death: a closed cohort study. Gastrointest Endosc. 2012;76:110–7.

Martel M, Barkun AN, Menard C, et al. Split-dose preparations are superior to day-before bowel cleansing regimens: a meta-analysis. Gastroenterology. 2015;149:79–88.

Matsuda T, Ono A, Sekiguchi M, et al. Advances in image enhancement in colonoscopy for detection of adenomas. Nat Rev Gastroenterol Hepatol. 2017;14:305–14.

Nagorni A, Bjelakovic G, Petrovic B. Narrow band imaging versus conventional white light colonoscopy for the detection of colorectal polyps. Cochrane Database Syst Rev. 2012;1:Cd008361.

Ng SC, Tsoi KK, Hirai HW, et al. The efficacy of cap-assisted colonoscopy in polyp detection and cecal intubation: a meta-analysis of randomized controlled trials. Am J Gastroenterol. 2012;107:1165–73.

Nishihara R, Wu K, Lochhead P, et al. Long-term colorectal-cancer incidence and mortality after lower endoscopy. N Engl J Med. 2013;369:1095–105.

Omata F, Ohde S, Deshpande GA, et al. Image-enhanced, chromo, and cap-assisted colonoscopy for improving adenoma/neoplasia detection rate: a systematic review and meta-analysis. Scand J Gastroenterol. 2014;49:222–37.

Peng L, Weigl K, Boakye D, et al. Risk scores for predicting advanced colorectal neoplasia in the average-risk population: a systematic review and meta-analysis. Am J Gastroenterol. 2018;113:1788–800.

Pox CP, Altenhofen L, Brenner H, et al. Efficacy of a nationwide screening colonoscopy program for colorectal cancer. Gastroenterology. 2012;142:1460–7.

Quintero E, Castells A, Bujanda L, et al. Colonoscopy versus fecal immunochemical testing in colorectal-cancer screening. N Engl J Med. 2012;366:697–706.

Reumkens A, Rondagh EJ, Bakker CM, et al. Post-colonoscopy complications: a systematic review, time trends, and meta-analysis of population-based studies. Am J Gastroenterol. 2016;111:1092–101.

Rex DK, Schoenfeld PS, Cohen J, et al. Quality indicators for colonoscopy. Gastrointest Endosc. 2015;81:31–53.

Rex DK, Repici A, Gross SA, et al. High-definition colonoscopy versus Endocuff versus EndoRings versus full-spectrum endoscopy for adenoma detection at colonoscopy: a multicenter randomized trial. Gastrointest Endosc. 2018;88:335–44.

Saito H, Kudo SE, Takahashi N, Yamamoto S, Kodama K, Nagata K, Mizota Y, Ishida F, Ohashi Y. Efficacy of screening using annual fecal immunochemical test alone versus combined with one-time colonoscopy in reducing colorectal cancer mortality: the Akita Japan population-based colonoscopy screening trial (Akita pop-colon trial). Int J Colorectal Dis. 2020;35(5):933-939. https://doi.org/10.1007/s00384-020-03518-w. Epub 2020 Feb 7. PMID: 32034490.

Schoen RE, Pinsky PF, Weissfeld JL, et al. Colorectal-cancer incidence and mortality with screening flexible sigmoidoscopy. N Engl J Med. 2012;366:2345–57.

Schreuders EH, Ruco A, Rabeneck L, et al. Colorectal cancer screening: a global overview of existing programmes. Gut. 2015;64:1637–49.

Segnan N, Armaroli P, Bonelli L, et al. Once-only sigmoidoscopy in colorectal cancer screening: follow-up findings of the Italian randomized controlled trial—SCORE. J Natl Cancer Inst. 2011;103:1310–22.

Sekiguchi M, Kakugawa Y, Matsumoto M, et al. A scoring model for predicting advanced colorectal neoplasia in a screened population of asymptomatic Japanese individuals. J Gastroenterol. 2018;53:1109–19.

Sekiguchi M, Otake Y, Kakugawa Y, et al. Incidence of advanced colorectal neoplasia in individuals with untreated diminutive colorectal adenomas diagnosed by magnifying image-enhanced endoscopy. Am J Gastroenterol. 2019;114:964–73.

Showa University Northern Yokohama Hospital. Randomized controlled trial to evaluate the effectiveness of total colonoscopy in colorectal cancer screening. UMIN000001980. n.d.. https://upload.umin.ac.jp/cgi-open-bin/ctr_e/ctr_view.cgi?recptno=R000002416. Accessed 8 Aug 2019.

Sung JJY, Wong MCS, Lam TYT, et al. A modified colorectal screening score for prediction of advanced neoplasia: a prospective study of 5744 subjects. J Gastroenterol Hepatol. 2018;33:187–94.

U.S. Department of Veterans Affairs. Colonoscopy versus fecal immunochemical test in reducing mortality from colorectal cancer (CONFIRM). n.d.. ClinicalTrials.gov. https://clinicaltrials.gov/ct2/show/NCT01239082. Accessed 8 Aug 2019.

Uppsala University Hospital. Colonoscopy and FIT as colorectal cancer screening test in the average risk population. ClinicalTrials.gov. https://clinicaltrials.gov/ct2/show/NCT02078804. Accessed 8 Aug 2019.

Wang L, Mannalithara A, Singh G, et al. Low rates of gastrointestinal and non-gastrointestinal complications for screening or surveillance colonoscopies in a population-based study. Gastroenterology. 2018;154:540–55.

Westwood DA, Alexakis N, Connor SJ. Transparent cap-assisted colonoscopy versus standard adult colonoscopy: a systematic review and meta-analysis. Dis Colon Rectum. 2012;55:218–25.

Winawer SJ, Zauber AG, Ho MN, et al. Prevention of colorectal cancer by colonoscopic polypectomy. The National Polyp study workgroup. N Engl J Med. 1993;329:1977–81.

Wong MC, Ching JY, Ng S, et al. The discriminatory capability of existing scores to predict advanced colorectal neoplasia: a prospective colonoscopy study of 5,899 screening participants. Sci Rep. 2016;6:20080.

Yeoh KG, Ho KY, Chiu HM, Asia-Pacific Working Group on Colorectal Cancer, et al. The Asia-Pacific colorectal screening score: a validated tool that stratifies risk for colorectal advanced neoplasia in asymptomatic Asian subjects. Gut. 2011;60:1236–41.

Zauber AG, Lansdorp-Vogelaar I, Knudsen AB, et al. Evaluating test strategies for colorectal cancer screening: a decision analysis for the U.S. preventive services task force. Ann Intern Med. 2008;149:659–69.

Zauber AG, Winawer SJ, O'Brien MJ, et al. Colonoscopic polypectomy and long-term prevention of colorectal-cancer deaths. N Engl J Med. 2012;366:687–96.

Han-Mo Chiu and Li-Chun Chang

Abstract

Noninvasive colorectal cancer (CRC) screening test enables selection of subjects at risk of significant neoplasm (cancer or advanced adenoma) from a large target screening population. It may, therefore, reduce the demand for colonoscopy, increase the likelihood of detecting significant neoplasm at colonoscopy and improve the efficiency of screening. Many population screening programs use noninvasive screening tests, such as guaiac fecal occult blood test or fecal immunochemical test as a primary screening test. Some important issues should be carefully considered when appraising a noninvasive test for screening: (1) test performance (sensitivity and specificity); (2) acceptance of the test by the public; and (3) cost of the test. In this chapter, two main categories of noninvasive test—stool- and blood-based screening tests, will be introduced and discussed based on current evidence.

Keywords

Screening · Colorectal cancer (CRC) · Fecal immunochemical test (FIT) · Fecal occult blood test (FOBT) · Blood-based screening test · Sensitivity · Specificity

5.1 Introduction

Screening for colorectal cancer (CRC) is concerned with many aspects of demands, including manpower demand such as public health workers, healthcare professionals, and laboratory staffs; clinical infrastructures such as endoscopy service and medical management of screening-detected neoplasms (adenoma or cancer); and sustained administrative and funding support. Currently, colonoscopy is deemed as the most accurate examination in detecting colorectal neoplasms, which has sensitivity of higher than 95% for detecting both advanced adenoma and invasive cancers. It also has the advantage of being able to resect neoplastic lesions that detected during examination thus it is nowadays not only used as a diagnostic exam but also as a primary screening tool in some countries (Lieberman et al. 2000). Its effectiveness in reducing CRC mortality and incidence has been demonstrated in several cohort studies (Nishihara et al. 2013; Zauber et al. 2012; Kahi et al. 2009; Jacob et al.

H.-M. Chiu (✉) · L.-C. Chang
Department of Internal Medicine, National Taiwan University Hospital, Taipei, Taiwan

Department of Internal Medicine, College of Medicine, National Taiwan University, Taipei, Taiwan
e-mail: hanmochiu@ntu.edu.tw;
lichunchang@ntu.edu.tw

© Springer Nature Singapore Pte Ltd. 2021
H.-M. Chiu, H.-H. Chen (eds.), *Colorectal Cancer Screening*,
https://doi.org/10.1007/978-981-15-7482-5_5

2012; Brenner et al. 2011). Nevertheless, if we consider the prevalence of neoplasm (0.2–0.3% for invasive cancer, 5–10% for advanced adenoma and 30–40% for adenoma) in the general population of screening age (i.e. 50–75 years in most of the screening programs), nearly 60–70% of the exams would be negative for neoplasm if colonoscopy is used as a primary screening tool for the targeted screening population. Adding to the fact that not all adenoma (especially diminutive or small ones) would eventually progress into invasive cancer, and the high invasiveness and high-cost characteristics of colonoscopy, it would be most ideal if we can select subjects at higher risk of advanced neoplasm from a large population by using a triage test (Inadomi et al. 2012; Quintero et al. 2012). Such a triage test should have the characteristics of low-cost, high accuracy, and high acceptance by the public.

Using the noninvasive test as the primary screening tool to select subjects at risk of sig-

nificant colorectal neoplasm can increase the likelihood of detecting significant neoplasm at colonoscopy (Fig. 5.1). For example, the positivity rate of FIT in population screening, which is the major determinant for colonoscopy demand, usually ranges from 4 to 10% (Chiu et al. 2015; Zorzi et al. 2015; Moss et al. 2017). This means colonoscopy capacity that required in FIT screening program is much lower than that in the colonoscopy-based screening settings. It can therefore remarkably reduce the colonoscopy demand thereby improve the efficiency of screening and reduce colonoscopy-related cost and unnecessary complications.

When choosing a primary screening test for population screening, several issues have to be carefully considered:

- *Test sensitivity*: High test sensitivity enables better detection of advanced neoplasm (advanced adenoma and cancer) and reduces

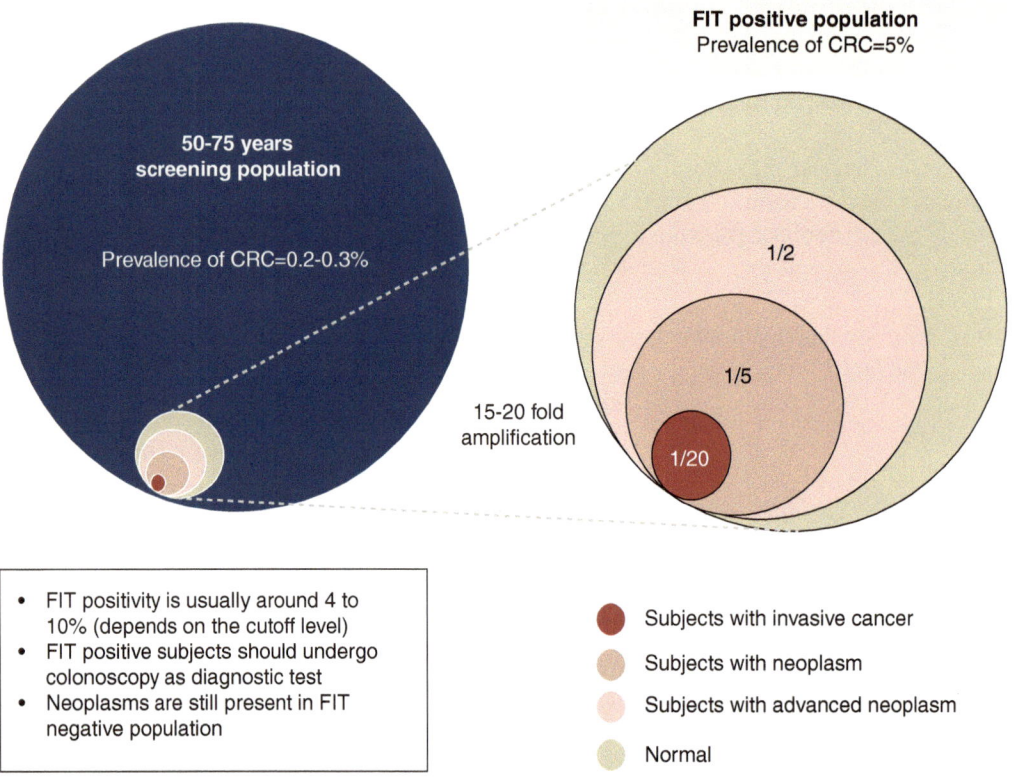

Fig. 5.1 Diagrams demonstrating how noninvasive screening test identifies high-risk subjects from large screening population (use FIT screening as an example)

missed lesions, leading to a higher screening effectiveness.

- *Test specificity*: High specificity can reduce the number of false-positive tests hence reduce the likelihood of unnecessary colonoscopy (negative finding for neoplasm at diagnostic colonoscopy) thereby improves the efficiency, colonoscopy-related complication, and the cost pertaining to diagnostic examination (i.e. colonoscopy or other imaging exams).
- *Positivity rate:* Positivity rate is not only associated with sensitivity and specificity of the test but is also affected by disease prevalence. High positivity rate is associated with increased workload of public health workers, medical and paramedical staffs, diagnostic examination demand and its related cost, and affects screening efficiency as well.
- *Cost*: Cost is another important consideration and may affect screening-related finance. This is extraordinarily important when the funding is constrained. In some screening program, screening test or diagnostic examination is only partially subsidized therefore screening participation would be affected if out-of-pocket expense pertaining to such cost is too high.
- *Public acceptance*: High screening test performance is not a guarantee of high screening participation by the public. Only if uptake of the CRC screening test is high then we can achieve a high detection rate for advanced neoplasms.

Currently, stool-based test, either guaiac occult blood test (gFOBT) or fecal immunochemical test (FIT), fit the above-mentioned characteristics (though the degree is different) and its effectiveness in reducing CRC mortality by screening has been proven in previous randomized controlled trials (gFOBT) or large cohort studies (gFOBT and FIT) (Chiu et al. 2015; Zorzi et al. 2015; Hewitson et al. 2008). In resource-limited regions, population mass screening with colonoscopy may not be a practical option, and strategies using non-invasive triage test to select high-risk population should be considered. In most of the government funded screening program, stool-based test (gFOBT or FIT) is used as the primary

screening tool. In contrast, colonoscopy was applied mostly in opportunistic screening setting in U.S. or in some organized screening programs such as in Germany and Poland (Schreuders et al. 2015).

One very important consideration of choosing screening test, as mentioned previously, is the preference by the public. The impact of preference on neoplasm is remarkable, if we look at the following formula:

$$\text{Detection} = \text{Screening test sensitivity} \times \text{screening partcipation}$$

From this formula, it is not difficult to understand that test sensitivity is not the sole major determinant of neoplasm detection in population screening because even with very high sensitivity, lesion detection would be low if the public acceptance of the screening test is very low. The following examples demonstrate how important screening participation is. In a Spanish randomized controlled trial comparing colonoscopy or FIT as the primary screening tool, the rate of participation was higher in the FIT group than in the colonoscopy group (34.2% vs. 24.6%, $P < 0.001$). As a consequence, with such 10% difference in screening participation, there was no significant difference in detection rate for CRC (0.1% in both colonoscopy and FIT screening arms, odds ratio = 0.99; 95% confidence interval = 0.61–1.64; $P = 0.99$) (Quintero et al. 2012). Even within the stool-based screening tests, the difference in screening uptake may exist and affects neoplasm detection. In a Dutch study by van Rossum et al., it was demonstrated that FIT had 12.7% significantly higher screening participation rate ($P < 0.01$) compared with gFOBT, leading to a higher detection rate for CRC and advanced adenoma (van Rossum et al. 2008). This was mainly caused by adsorbing the need for dietary restriction prior to sample collection by FIT and its user-friendly design of stool collection tube thereby improved the compliance of the screening population, leading to higher detection of advanced neoplasm.

There also exists difference in preference toward screening tests among different population. One US randomized trial involving different ethnicities (Caucasians, African Americans, Latinos, and Asians), participants who were recommended colonoscopy completed screening at a significantly lower rate (38%) than participants who were recommended FOBT (67%) (*P* < 0.001) or given a choice between FOBT or colonoscopy (69%) (*P* < 0.001) and nonwhite participants (Latino or Asian) adhered more often to FOBT, while white participants adhered more often to colonoscopy (Inadomi et al. 2012). Collectively, it is therefore important to take into account all the abovementioned issues, when considering a screening test. Not only screening provider but also public perspectives are important because they may affect screening participation and hence largely impact on neoplasm detection and resultant effectiveness of screening.

5.2   Stool-Based Tests

5.2.1   Guaiac FOBT

Guaiac FOBT (gFOBT) is one of the earliest stool tests used for CRC screening. Detection of blood by gFOBT is dependent on heme in stools. When hydrogen peroxide is added to the stool sample during analysis, heme reacts with the hydrogen peroxide developer to oxidize guaiac, resulting in a color change to blue (Fig. 5.2). As the determination of positivity relies on manual operation and subjective judgment of the color change, quality assurance is difficult and variations in reading among laboratory staffs have been the major concerns of gFOBT. Moreover, gFOBT is also reported to be affected by animal food products (e.g., beef, pork, lamb, and processed foods containing these meats) because they contain heme. Some programs advise avoiding those foods before stool sampling to reduce false-positive test but this may adversely affect screening participation because usually 3–6 stool samples are required for gFOBT.

Given its effectiveness being proven in previous randomized trials with pooled effectiveness of 16% in reducing CRC mortality in a meta-analysis, its effectiveness on CRC incidence is rather low because the sensitivity of gFOBT for

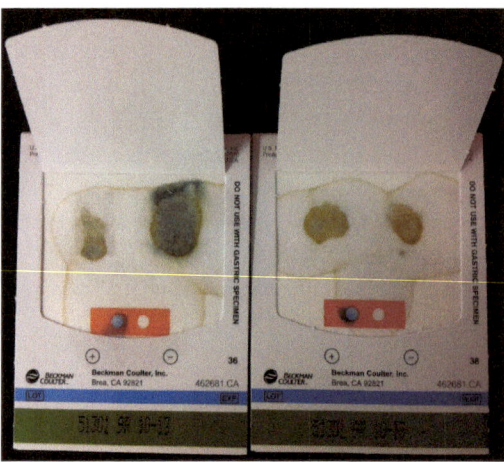

Fig. 5.2 Guaiac-based fecal occult blood test card. The patient recovers stool from the toilet bowl using a wooden applicator, smears a small portion of the stool sample onto two windows of the card, and closes the cover. Usually, this is done on three successive days (more days in some programs), and the cards are mailed to the laboratory for testing. There is little degradation of reactive heme in the dry, smeared specimens over a period of 1 week (fewer than 15% of samples). Appearance of unequivocal blue color, of any intensity, within 10 s, is considered a positive test, which usually remains stable for at least 1 min

advanced adenoma is rather low (Hewitson et al. 2008). Rehydrated gFOBT has higher sensitivity but at the cost of much higher positivity rate with resultant lower specificity compared with nonhydrated FBOT (Levin et al. 1997). Though gradually being replaced by FIT, gFOBT is currently still used in many screening programs, such as in the United Kingdom, Canada (Ontario and Manitoba), Finland, and Croatia (Schreuders et al. 2015).

5.2.2   Fecal Immunochemical Test

FIT is less likely affected by diet because it is an immunoassay specific for human hemoglobin. Typically, only one or two stool samples are required and dietary restriction is obviated for FIT testing, and adding the user-friendly design of spatula and stool sample collection tube (Fig. 5.3), its acceptance by the public is much higher than gFOBT thereby contributing to

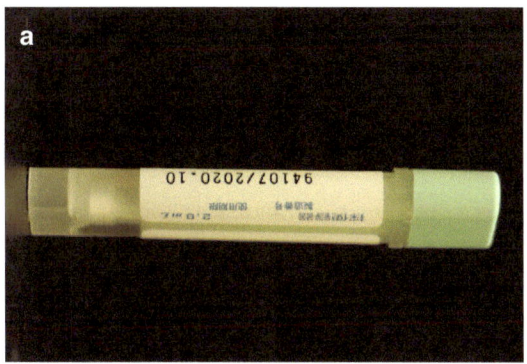
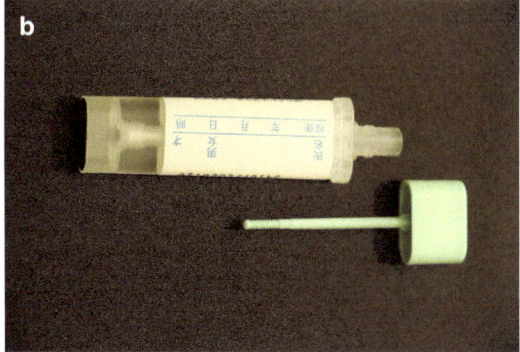

Fig. 5.3 Fecal immunochemical test. (**a**) External appearance of a FIT kit. (**b**) Test-wand integrated with cap (left) and sample collection tube (right). The groove at the tip of the test-wand may facilitate a fixed amount of stool sampling. The sample buffer solution in the collection tube included guarantees optimum stabilization of the hemoglobin in the sample from collection to analysis in the laboratory (7 days at room temperature, 28 days at 2–8 °C)

higher neoplasm detection (Moss et al. 2017; van Rossum et al. 2008).

FIT is currently the most popular primary screening test worldwide, especially in government-funded programs because they can significantly constrain the demand for colonoscopy and enable high-throughput sample handling (Schreuders et al. 2015). Though only gFOBT was proven to be effective in reducing CRC mortality by randomized trials, FIT has the advantages of superior screening uptake, higher sensitivity to early CRC and advanced adenoma, and higher specificity as compared with gFOBT. It is nowadays gradually replacing gFOBT and becomes the most popular primary screening test (Hewitson et al. 2008; van Rossum et al. 2008). Its effectiveness and cost-effectiveness in reducing CRC mortality or incidence is considered as higher than gFOBT according to modeling studies (Zauber et al. 2008; Knudsen et al. 2016).

Quantitative FIT, for which positive cutoff is adjustable, can help the screening organizer to determine the optimal cutoff of FIT based on the regional colonoscopy capacity, prevalence of advanced colorectal neoplasm (CRC and advanced adenoma) and healthcare cost (Chen et al. 2007). Whilst determining positive cutoff, evaluation from different aspects is indispensable. Taking Taiwan CRC screening program as an example, before the launch of the nationwide screening program, a receiver operating characteristic (ROC) analysis based on the results (screening participation rate, diagnostic examination rate, neoplasm detection rate, etc.) of pilot study and a cost-effectiveness analysis taking into account the local medical care cost were conducted. The results suggested that 20 μg hemoglobin/g of feces was the optimal positive cutoff in Taiwanese population (Chen et al. 2007; Yang et al. 2006). Qualitative FIT, which uses fixed cutoff, is also used in some population screening programs. A study from Korean screening program revealed that the positivity rate of the qualitative FIT was around three times higher than that of the quantitative FIT but the likelihood of detecting of "suspicious cancer and cancer" versus "normal" of the quantitative FIT was about three times higher than that of the qualitative FIT (Park et al. 2012). Though multiple brands of qualitative FIT with possibly different performances were used in Korean programs, its performance seems different from that of FIT even with the same cutoff as claimed by the manufacturers.

The sensitivity of FIT for invasive CRC is around 80% and advanced adenoma around 30%, both are much lower than colonoscopy. Therefore repeat FIT at fixed intervals is required to detect neoplasm missed at previous screening round or newly developed ones (Lee et al. 2014). One or two years are the most widely applied screening intervals for FIT, which is based on the sojourn time for an advanced adenoma to progress into invasive cancer (estimated to be around 3 years).

Several programs have reported the effectiveness of FIT screening in reducing CRC mortality or even CRC incidence (Chiu et al. 2015; Zorzi et al. 2015; Giorgi Rossi et al. 2015; Levin et al. 2018). FIT can be similar in effectiveness to colonoscopy when used in a consistent, programmatic way to screen for CRC given a high adherence to regular screening. Its cost-effectiveness, based on the modeling study by the United States Preventive Services Task Force (USPSTF), is also close to that of colonoscopy-based screening if adherence to FIT screening over time is good (Knudsen et al. 2016).

The limitations of FIT screening are several-fold. First, its sensitivity for detection of neoplasm is stage dependent. Though the overall sensitivity of FIT for CRC was reported to be around 80%, such a figure is actually the pooled result of sensitivity of 60% for stage 1 CRC and 90–95% for CRC of stage 2 or higher (Lee et al. 2014). Such deficit of FIT in detecting early-stage CRC may cause interval cancers after a false negative FIT and affect the screening effectiveness. Secondly, FIT has lower sensitivity for proximal neoplasm. Previous studies have demonstrated that FIT has a significantly lower sensitivity for proximal colon cancer or advanced adenoma (Wong et al. 2015; Chiu et al. 2013). It is reasonable to speculate that a more advanced degree of hemoglobin degradation of small amounts of blood to originate from proximally located lesions during bowel passage and result in false-negative results of FIT. A study by Chang et al. also demonstrated that FIT has much lower sensitivity for sessile serrated polyps, which are mainly located at proximal colon and have been demonstrated to consist of more than 20% of all CRC, compared with that for conventional adenoma (Chang et al. 2017). Nevertheless, stool-based tests are basically designed to be applied annually or biennially, therefore, neoplasms not being detected in previous rounds are theoretically still possible to be detected subsequently and at a curable stage. To deal with this problem, several strategies may be taken, including shortening of inter-screening intervals, increasing stool sample numbers, and lowering the cutoff for determining FIT positivity. These approaches may speed up or increase

chances for detecting cancers at a curable or precancerous stage, but on the other hand may increase the demand for colonoscopy and put stress on the currently constrained colonoscopy capacity. Further study is warranted.

5.2.3 Multi-target Stool DNA Test

The multi-target stool DNA test not only detects the trace amounts of human hemoglobin in the stool (multi-target stool DNA test also contains FIT), but it also looks for certain specific DNA changes and mutations found in CRC or adenoma. Cells exfoliated from precancerous and cancerous lesions with these mutations often shed DNA biomarkers into the stool, where this test can detect them (11 distinct molecular biomarkers in the stool sample, including seven DNA mutation biomarkers, two DNA methylation biomarkers, hemoglobin, and also β-actin as a control for human DNA), therefore indicating the presence of precancerous colorectal polyps or cancer.

The study by Imperiale et al. involving 9989 subjects revealed that the sensitivity for detecting CRC was 92.3% with DNA testing and 73.8% with FIT ($P = 0.002$). The sensitivity for detecting advanced precancerous lesions was 42.4% with DNA testing and 23.8% with FIT ($P < 0.001$). The rate of detection of polyps with high-grade dysplasia was 69.2% with DNA testing and 46.2% with FIT ($P = 0.004$); the rates of detection of serrated sessile polyps measuring 1 cm or more were 42.4% and 5.1%, respectively ($P < 0.001$). Specificity of multi-target DNA testing was lower than FIT (86.6% vs. 94.9%, $P < 0.01$) among those with non-advanced or negative findings (Imperiale et al. 2014). Given the significantly higher performance than FIT, there exits several barriers for its use in organized large-scale screening programs. They include a very high cost (more than 500 USD, which is even much higher than colonoscopy in many countries), and a more tedious stool sampling process and increased laboratory workload. Its acceptance by the public is largely unknown, especially when the abovementioned barriers are taken into consideration. The low specificity may also increase the colonoscopy demand and the "genetically-positive" test results may lead to inappropriate additional testing such as repeat colonoscopy or even PET/CT/MRI to search for other digestive cancers that may give rise to a positive DNA test.

Currently, US FDA approves (approved in 2014) 3-yearly multi-target stool DNA test for CRC screening but the cost-effectiveness was, however, inferior to either direct colonoscopy or FIT screening according to the modeling study by Knudsen et al. (2016).

5.2.4 Other Stool Biomarkers

Alternations in the gut microbial composition are associated with CRC and its precancerous neoplasia, with an increased abundance of *Fusobacterium* and other bacteria. Fecal microbial biomarkers were therefore considered as useful for CRC screening (Yu et al. 2017; Nakatsu et al. 2015; Feng et al. 2015). A study by Wong et al. measured relative abundance of *Fusobacterium nucleatum* (*Fn*), *Peptostreptococcus anaerobius*, and *Parvimonas micra* by quantitative PCR in 309 subjects, including 104 patients with CRC, 103 patients with advanced adenoma and 102 controls. The results showed that abundance was higher for all three individual markers in patients with CRC than controls ($P < 0.001$), and for marker *Fn* in patients with advanced adenoma than controls ($P = 0.022$). The marker *Fn*, when combined with FIT, showed superior sensitivity (92.3% vs. 73.1%, $P < 0.001$) and area under the receiver-operating characteristic curve (AUC) (0.95 vs. 0.86, $P < 0.001$) than stand-alone FIT in detecting CRC in the same patient cohort. From the result of this study, though Fn alone had a comparable performance with that of FIT (AUC = 0.83 vs. 0.86, $P > 0.05$), the most prominent gain was observed when the marker *Fn* was used in combination with FIT, resulting in a detection leap of 20% without significantly sacrificing its specificity. Fn detected neoplasms that were missed by FIT thus was considered as compensatory to FIT (Wong et al. 2017). Future challenge of applying microbial biomarkers in

CRC screening would be its validation in large and different ethnic groups, subjects with different dietary habits, standardization of stool sampling and processing, testing public acceptance in screening population, identifying potential confounders to such test, and development of a high throughput platform for handling a large number of stool samples in screening settings.

5.3 Blood-Based Tests

There are several blood-based tests for CRC screening being developed and tested in clinical settings. They include circulating methylated DNA markers, miRNA markers, nucleosome markers, and γ-interferon released by activated NK cells (Table 5.1). Some studies have demonstrated that blood-based screening tests had a high acceptance by subjects who were not compliant to colonoscopy or stool-based screening hence were considered as being able to fill the gap of insufficient test uptake in the screening program (Liles et al. 2017; Adler et al. 2014).

DNA methylation is assumed to be an early event in tumorigenesis and has therefore been proposed as a potential marker for the detection of cancers at an early stage as epigenetic changes occur at a higher frequency compared with genetic changes. Many screening tests measuring the methylated circulating tumor DNA was therefore developed for CRC screening (Xue et al. 2015). Of those studies investigating such markers for CRC screening, some demonstrated that blood-based screening test could have significantly higher acceptance by the public compared with currently used stool-based tests or endoscopic exams. Adler et al. demonstrated in their study that when screening colonoscopy was offered, only 63 of 172 subjects were compliant (37%) and 106 of the 109 subjects who declined colonoscopy accepted an alternative non-invasive method (97%) and 90 of them selected the Septin 9 blood test (83%), whereas 16 selected a stool test (15%), and 3 refused any test (3%). The reasons for choosing blood test included convenience of an office draw, overall convenience, and less time-consuming procedure (Adler et al. 2014).

Table 5.1 Summary of blood test developed for CRC screening

Biomarker	Case number	Sample	Sensitivity %	Specificity %	References
miRNA					
miR-17-3p	205	Plasma	64	70	Ng et al. (2009)
miR-18a	164	Plasma	73.1	79.1	Zhang et al. (2013)
miR-20a	179	Plasma	46	73.4	Chen et al. (2015)
miR-21	71	Plasma	90	90	Kanaan et al. (2012)
miR-29a	159	Plasma	69	89.1	Huang et al. (2010)
miR-92	205	Plasma	89	70	Ng et al. (2009)
miR-96	287	Plasma	65.4	73.3	Sun et al. (2016)
miR-106a	179	Plasma	74	44.4	Chen et al. (2015)
miR-200c	164	Plasma	64.1	73.3	Zhang et al. (2013)
miR-210	370	Serum	74.6	73.5	Wang et al. (2017)
miR-221	140	Plasma	86	41	Pu et al. (2010)
miR-372	195	Serum	81.9	73.3	Yu et al. (2016)
miR-24	241	Plasma	78.4	83.9	Fang et al. (2015)
miR-29b	305	Serum	61.4	72.5	Li et al. (2015)
miR-194	110	Serum	72	80	Basati et al. (2016)
miR-320a	241	Plasma	92.8	73.1	Fang et al. (2015)
miR-375	140	Plasma	76.9	64.6	Xu et al. (2014)
miR-423-5p	241	Plasma	91.9	70.8	Fang et al. (2015)
miR-601	71	Serum	69.2	72.4	Wang et al. (2012)
miR-760	71	Serum	80	72.4	Wang et al. (2012)
Cell-free DNA					
Alu 115	281	Serum	69.2	99.1	Hao et al. (2014)
H1C1	60	Plasma	54.6	64.5	Cassinotti et al. (2012)
MDG1	60	Plasma	54.6	64.5	Cassinotti et al. (2012)
Septin 9	144	Plasma	90	88	Warren et al. (2011)
Septin 9	7941	Plasma	48.2	91.5	Church et al. (2014)
BCAT1/IKZF1	2105	Plasma	66	94	Pedersen et al. (2015a)
Nucleosome					
Nucleosome panel	42	Serum	74	90	Rahier et al. (2017)
NK cell activity					
ϒ-interferon	872	Supernatant	87	60.8	Jobin et al. (2017)

One randomized trial by Liles et al. revealed that of those 413 subjects randomized to either FIT or blood-based test, 99.5% (CI95: 97.3%–100%) of participants in the blood test arm and 88.1% (CI95: 83.0%–91.8%) of participants in the FIT arm completed the offered test yielding a difference of 11.4% (CI95: 6.9%–15.9%, $P < 0.001$) (Liles et al. 2017). A study using methylated *BCAT1* and *IKZF1* genes test identified 85 of 129 CRC cases (sensitivity of 66%, 95% CI: 57–74). For CRC stages I–IV, respective positivity rates were 38% (95% CI: 21–58), 69% (95% CI: 53–82), 73% (95% CI: 56–85), and 94% (95% CI: 70–100) (Pedersen et al. 2015a, b). Another

type of blood-based test measuring NK cell activity via measuring the amount of Interferon-gamma (IFN-γ) secreted after artificially activating NK cells in the blood was also developed for CRC screening. In an open-label, prospective, cross-sectional study of 872 high-risk subjects in Canada, the NK cell activity test identified subjects with CRC with 87.0% sensitivity, 60.8% specificity, a positive predictive value of 5.7%, and a negative predictive value of 99.4%. The odds ratio for detection of CRC in subjects with low NK cell activity vs. subjects with higher NK cell activity was 10.3 (95% CI, 3.03–34.9) (Jobin et al. 2017).

Nevertheless, blood-based testing has higher public acceptance, none of the currently existent organized screening programs apply such an approach for population CRC screening mainly because its insufficient performance compared with currently used frontline screening test such as FIT, lacking relevant evidences (screening uptake, test performance, and effect on incidence or mortality reduction) in a large screening population. After a preliminary study in a hospital setting, the tests are still needed to be tested in "real screening population" not only to test their performance in real-world setting with changeable environments (temperatures, sample preservation, etc.) and populations (ethnicity, age groups, etc.) but also the acceptance by the public over multiple screening rounds, its effectiveness or cost-effectiveness. Taking Septin 9 test as an example, in an earlier study, Warren et al. reported the encouraging overall sensitivity of Septin 9 test for CRC of 90% (95% CI, 77.4% to 96.3%) and specificity of 88% (95% CI, 79.6% to 93.7%) (Warren et al. 2011). In a latter study in large screening population (7941 subjects), however, Church et al. demonstrated that overall sensitivity of Septin 9 test for CRC was 48.2% (95% CI 32.4% to 63.6%); for CRC stages I–IV, values were 35.0%, 63.0%, 46.0%, and 77.4%, respectively. The specificity was 91.5% (95% CI 89.7% to 93.1%) and the sensitivity for advanced adenomas was low (11.2%) (Church et al. 2014). Such a low sensitivity for CRC confined its use for only those who have history of declining other CRC screening tests such as colonoscopy, flexible sigmoidoscopy, FIT, or gFOBT. In a modeling study by Ladabaum et al., though Septin 9 seems to be effective and cost-effective compared with no screening, to be cost-effective compared with currently established strategies (colonoscopy, sigmoidoscopy, FIT, gFOBT, and combination of flexible sigmoidoscopy with FIT or gFOBT), Septin 9 test or blood-based biomarkers with similar test performance characteristics would need to achieve substantially higher uptake and adherence rates than the alternatives.

Nevertheless, blood-based test seems promising in filling the deficit of current CRC screening approaches, several barriers should be cleared before becoming a frontline screening test in large-scale screening settings. First, many of the studies are not conducted in a real screening population. If we look into those literatures, some studies cohorts are enriched by more advanced stage CRCs leading to a higher sensitivity of the tests. In real asymptomatic screening population, however, the majority of the CRCs are early-stage ones, therefore, good performance in the aforementioned hospital-based or case-control studies do not guarantee a good performance in the real screening settings. Second, proof of a test being able to detect cancer is not the same as proof that the test can reduce disease-specific mortality. CRCs are heterogeneous cancers with distinct survival in relation to different biology (CRCs have arisen via serrated pathway vs. traditional adenoma carcinoma sequence) therefore high sensitivity to CRCs may not necessarily lead to better survival. Third, reduction of CRC incidence by screening tests is mainly attributable to detection of the precancerous lesions. Currently, most of the blood-based screening tests have low sensitivity to detect adenoma or advanced adenoma (most of them had a sensitivity of around 10%), which need further improvement. Fourth, although blood-based screening should be used for individuals eligible for but nonadherent with other screening methods (stool-based test or endoscopy), it is possible that the test will undergo indication drift—in both directions (Parikh and Prasad 2016). Availability of a blood test may increase CRC screening among those who should not be screened. In the other direction, given the convenience of blood testing, patients who arc appropriate candidates for endoscopy may wish to first be tested with this assay in lieu or in advance of endoscopy.

Along with more molecular ways to detect CRC being discovered, the medical community has the obligation to carefully consider the standard for integrating these markers as screening tests using the same standard for appraisal of currently used screening tests (e.g., randomized trial or large cohort study to evaluate stool-based or endoscopy-based screening modalities).

References

Adler A, Geiger S, Keil A, et al. Improving compliance to colorectal cancer screening using blood and stool based tests in patients refusing screening colonoscopy in Germany. BMC Gastroenterol. 2014;14:183.

Basati G, Razavi AE, Pakzad I, et al. Circulating levels of the miRNAs, miR-194, and miR-29b, as clinically useful biomarkers for colorectal cancer. Tumour Biol. 2016;37:1781–8.

Brenner H, Chang-Claude J, Seiler CM, et al. Protection from colorectal cancer after colonoscopy: a population-based, case-control study. Ann Intern Med. 2011;154:22–30.

Cassinotti E, Melson J, Liggett T, et al. DNA methylation patterns in blood of patients with colorectal cancer and adenomatous colorectal polyps. Int J Cancer. 2012;131:1153–7.

Chang LC, Shun CT, Hsu WF, et al. Fecal immunochemical test detects sessile serrated adenomas and polyps with a low level of sensitivity. Clin Gastroenterol Hepatol. 2017;15:872–9.

Chen LS, Liao CS, Chang SH, et al. Cost-effectiveness analysis for determining optimal cut-off of immunochemical faecal occult blood test for population-based colorectal cancer screening (KCIS 16). J Med Screen. 2007;14:191–9.

Chen WY, Zhao XJ, Yu ZF, et al. The potential of plasma miRNAs for diagnosis and risk estimation of colorectal cancer. Int J Clin Exp Pathol. 2015;8:7092–101.

Chiu HM, Lee YC, Tu CH, et al. Association between early stage colon neoplasms and false-negative results from the fecal immunochemical test. Clin Gastroenterol Hepatol. 2013;11:832-8 e1-2.

Chiu HM, Chen SL, Yen AM, et al. Effectiveness of fecal immunochemical testing in reducing colorectal cancer mortality from the one million Taiwanese screening program. Cancer. 2015;121:3221–9.

Church TR, Wandell M, Lofton-Day C, et al. Prospective evaluation of methylated SEPT9 in plasma for detection of asymptomatic colorectal cancer. Gut. 2014;63:317–25.

Fang Z, Tang J, Bai Y, et al. Plasma levels of microRNA-24, microRNA-320a, and microRNA-423-5p are potential biomarkers for colorectal carcinoma. J Exp Clin Cancer Res. 2015;34:86.

Feng Q, Liang S, Jia H, et al. Gut microbiome development along the colorectal adenoma-carcinoma sequence. Nat Commun. 2015;6:6528.

Giorgi Rossi P, Vicentini M, Sacchettini C, et al. Impact of screening program on incidence of colorectal cancer: a cohort study in Italy. Am J Gastroenterol. 2015;110:1359–66.

Hao TB, Shi W, Shen XJ, et al. Circulating cell-free DNA in serum as a biomarker for diagnosis and prognostic prediction of colorectal cancer. Br J Cancer. 2014;111:1482–9.

Hewitson P, Glasziou P, Watson E, et al. Cochrane systematic review of colorectal cancer screening using the fecal occult blood test (hemoccult): an update. Am J Gastroenterol. 2008;103:1541.

Huang Z, Huang D, Ni S, et al. Plasma microRNAs are promising novel biomarkers for early detection of colorectal cancer. Int J Cancer. 2010;127:118–26.

Imperiale TF, Ransohoff DF, Itzkowitz SH, et al. Multitarget stool DNA testing for colorectal-cancer screening. N Engl J Med. 2014;370:1287–97.

Inadomi JM, Vijan S, Janz NK, et al. Adherence to colorectal cancer screening: a randomized clinical trial of competing strategies. Arch Intern Med. 2012;172:575–82.

Jacob BJ, Moineddin R, Sutradhar R, et al. Effect of colonoscopy on colorectal cancer incidence and mortality: an instrumental variable analysis. Gastrointest Endosc. 2012;76:355–64. e1

Jobin G, Rodriguez-Suarez R, Betito K. Association between natural killer cell activity and colorectal cancer in high-risk subjects undergoing colonoscopy. Gastroenterology. 2017;153:980–7.

Kahi CJ, Imperiale TF, Juliar BE, et al. Effect of screening colonoscopy on colorectal cancer incidence and mortality. Clin Gastroenterol Hepatol. 2009;7:770–5. quiz 711

Kanaan Z, Rai SN, Eichenberger MR, et al. Plasma miR-21: a potential diagnostic marker of colorectal cancer. Ann Surg. 2012;256:544–51.

Knudsen AB, Zauber AG, Rutter CM, et al. Estimation of benefits, burden, and harms of colorectal cancer screening strategies: modeling study for the US preventive services task force. JAMA. 2016;315:2595–609.

Lee JK, Liles EG, Bent S, et al. Accuracy of fecal immunochemical tests for colorectal cancer: systematic review and meta-analysis. Ann Intern Med. 2014;160:171.

Levin B, Hess K, Johnson C. Screening for colorectal cancer. A comparison of 3 fecal occult blood tests. Arch Intern Med. 1997;157:970–6.

Levin TR, Corley DA, Jensen CD, et al. Effects of organized colorectal cancer screening on cancer incidence and mortality in a large community-based population. Gastroenterology. 2018;155:1383–91. e5

Li J, Liu Y, Wang C, et al. Serum miRNA expression profile as a prognostic biomarker of stage II/III colorectal adenocarcinoma. Sci Rep. 2015;5:12921.

Lieberman DA, Weiss DG, Bond JH, et al. Use of colonoscopy to screen asymptomatic adults for colorectal cancer. Veterans affairs cooperative study group 380. N Engl J Med. 2000;343:162–8.

Liles EG, Coronado GD, Perrin N, et al. Uptake of a colorectal cancer screening blood test is higher than of a fecal test offered in clinic: a randomized trial. Cancer Treat Res Commun. 2017;10:27–31.

Moss S, Mathews C, Day TJ, et al. Increased uptake and improved outcomes of bowel cancer screening with a faecal immunochemical test: results from a pilot study within the national screening programme in England. Gut. 2017;66:1631–44.

Nakatsu G, Li X, Zhou H, et al. Gut mucosal microbiome across stages of colorectal carcinogenesis. Nat Commun. 2015;6:8727.

Ng EK, Chong WW, Jin H, et al. Differential expression of microRNAs in plasma of patients with colorectal cancer: a potential marker for colorectal cancer screening. Gut. 2009;58:1375–81.

Nishihara R, Wu K, Lochhead P, et al. Long-term colorectal-cancer incidence and mortality after lower endoscopy. N Engl J Med. 2013;369:1095–105.

Parikh RB, Prasad V. Blood-based screening for colon cancer: a disruptive innovation or simply a disruption? JAMA. 2016;315:2519–20.

Park MJ, Choi KS, Lee YK, et al. A comparison of qualitative and quantitative fecal immunochemical tests in the Korean national colorectal cancer screening program. Scand J Gastroenterol. 2012;47:461–6.

Pedersen SK, Symonds EL, Baker RT, et al. Evaluation of an assay for methylated BCAT1 and IKZF1 in plasma for detection of colorectal neoplasia. BMC Cancer. 2015a;15:654.

Pedersen SK, Baker RT, McEvoy A, et al. A two-gene blood test for methylated DNA sensitive for colorectal cancer. PLoS One. 2015b;10:e0125041.

Pu XX, Huang GL, Guo HQ, et al. Circulating miR-221 directly amplified from plasma is a potential diagnostic and prognostic marker of colorectal cancer and is correlated with p53 expression. J Gastroenterol Hepatol. 2010;25:1674–80.

Quintero E, Castells A, Bujanda L, et al. Colonoscopy versus fecal immunochemical testing in colorectal-cancer screening. N Engl J Med. 2012;366:697–706.

Rahier JF, Druez A, Faugeras L, et al. Circulating nucleosomes as new blood-based biomarkers for detection of colorectal cancer. Clin Epigenetics. 2017;9:53.

Schreuders EH, Ruco A, Rabeneck L, et al. Colorectal cancer screening: a global overview of existing programmes. Gut. 2015;64:1637–49.

Sun Y, Liu Y, Cogdell D, et al. Examining plasma microRNA markers for colorectal cancer at different stages. Oncotarget. 2016;7:11434–49.

van Rossum LG, van Rijn AF, Laheij RJ, et al. Random comparison of guaiac and immunochemical fecal occult blood tests for colorectal cancer in a screening population. Gastroenterology. 2008;135:82–90.

Wang Q, Huang Z, Ni S, et al. Plasma miR-601 and miR-760 are novel biomarkers for the early detection of colorectal cancer. PLoS One. 2012;7:e44398.

Wang W, Qu A, Liu W, et al. Circulating miR-210 as a diagnostic and prognostic biomarker for colorectal cancer. Eur J Cancer Care (Engl). 2017;26

Warren JD, Xiong W, Bunker AM, et al. Septin 9 methylated DNA is a sensitive and specific blood test for colorectal cancer. BMC Med. 2011;9:133.

Wong MC, Ching JY, Chan VC, et al. Diagnostic accuracy of a qualitative fecal immunochemical test varies with location of neoplasia but not number of specimens. Clin Gastroenterol Hepatol. 2015;13:1472–9.

Wong SH, Kwong TNY, Chow TC, et al. Quantitation of faecal fusobacterium improves faecal immunochemical test in detecting advanced colorectal neoplasia. Gut. 2017;66:1441–8.

Xu L, Li M, Wang M, et al. The expression of microRNA-375 in plasma and tissue is matched in human colorectal cancer. BMC Cancer. 2014;14:714.

Xue M, Lai SC, Xu ZP, et al. Noninvasive DNA methylation biomarkers in colorectal cancer: a systematic review. J Dig Dis. 2015;16:699–712.

Yang KC, Liao CS, Chiu YH, et al. Colorectal cancer screening with faecal occult blood test within a multiple disease screening programme: an experience from Keelung, Taiwan. J Med Screen. 2006;13(Suppl 1):S8–13.

Yu J, Jin L, Jiang L, et al. Serum miR-372 is a diagnostic and prognostic biomarker in patients with early colorectal cancer. Anti Cancer Agents Med Chem. 2016;16:424–31.

Yu J, Feng Q, Wong SH, et al. Metagenomic analysis of faecal microbiome as a tool towards targeted non-invasive biomarkers for colorectal cancer. Gut. 2017;66:70–8.

Zauber AG, Lansdorp-Vogelaar I, Knudsen AB, et al. Evaluating test strategies for colorectal cancer screening: a decision analysis for the U.S. preventive services task force. Ann Intern Med. 2008;149:659–69.

Zauber AG, Winawer SJ, O'Brien MJ, et al. Colonoscopic polypectomy and long-term prevention of colorectal-cancer deaths. N Engl J Med. 2012;366:687–96.

Zhang GJ, Zhou T, Liu ZL, et al. Plasma miR-200c and miR-18a as potential biomarkers for the detection of colorectal carcinoma. Mol Clin Oncol. 2013;1:379–84.

Zorzi M, Fedeli U, Schievano E, et al. Impact on colorectal cancer mortality of screening programmes based on the faecal immunochemical test. Gut. 2015;64:784–90.

Health Information System in Population-Based Organized Service Screening for Colorectal Cancer

Sherry Yueh-Hsia Chiu and Sam Li-Sheng Chen

Abstract

Health information system supporting population-based organized service screening for colorectal cancer (CRC) is critically important for delivery, surveillance, and management of screening services in order to aid health professionals improving the quality assurance and enhancing the feasibility of evaluating the screening program.

Health information system embedded within a service-screening program include the infrastructure of the screening program, availability and comprehensiveness of screening data, and the sophisticated and precise data analysis with adjustment for potential biases. The infrastructure of the screening process includes three phases, pre-screening, screening, and post-screening phase. A centralized screening database linking various kinds of databases together from pre-screening phase is tremendously helpful for planning population-based organized service screening. During the screening phase, the key performance index should be collected for screening including the screening rate, positivity rate, diagnostic exam (colonoscopy) rate, positive predictive rate, detection rate, and interval cancer rate. Information provided from post-screening phase included surveillance of adenoma, effectiveness, and cost-effectiveness evaluation, and personalized strategies for colorectal cancer screening.

Systematic health information system for population-based organized service screening is conducive to evidence-based screening policy beyond randomized controlled trial.

Keywords

Screening infrastructure · Quality assurance indicator · Health information screening system

6.1 Integrated Information System for CRC Screening

The online information system facilities delivery, surveillance, and management of healthcare services in an organized service screening program. Such an infrastructure, as a part of the evaluation system, are of paramount importance in developing a health information system. A comprehensive health information system for colorectal cancer (CRC) screening is helpful for assisting health pro-

S. Y.-H. Chiu
Department of Health Care Management, College of Management, Chang Gung University, Taoyuan, Taiwan

S. L.-S. Chen (✉)
Research Center of Cancer Translational Medicine, Taipei Medical University, Taipei, Taiwan
e-mail: samchen@tmu.edu.tw

© Springer Nature Singapore Pte Ltd. 2021
H.-M. Chiu, H.-H. Chen (eds.), *Colorectal Cancer Screening*,
https://doi.org/10.1007/978-981-15-7482-5_6

fessionals in processing screening with quality assurance and evaluation, such information system should be able to aid health professionals and health decision makers in planning, delivering, managing, and evaluating the entire screening program.

6.2 Infrastructure and Workflow of Building up Information System

With the advent of online technology, a web-based solution combining data gathering and processing capabilities is the most popular approach. Application design in a server can be based on the ASP, HTML, DHTML, JavaScript, Java Applet technology, and SQL-based relational database. Web-based software programs are useful to facilitate the structure, process, and outcome for evaluation of screening, such as referral messages for those with positive screening tests to receive a confirmatory diagnosis without delay. Individual screen data further underpinning this model are transferred to centralized databases via the Internet. In Taiwan, around 3.8 million subjects aged 50–74 years have attended the biennial fecal immunochemical test (FIT) screening (Chiu et al. 2015). Information on organized features appertaining to screening, diagnosis, and outcomes after long-term follow-up are collected for the systematic evaluation. The proposed health information system for cancer screening is centered on modules that would allow for the computerization, process, update of screen data, and link with other registry data (e.g., population registry, cancer registry, and mortality).

The key performance index of a screening program, such as the screening rate, positivity rate, colonoscopy rate, positive predictive rate, detection rate, and interval cancer rate, are included in the system. The system allows for the information flow from different health services and geographical areas so as to monitor screening participation and every following step in the whole screening logistics. It also has an alert system to prevent delayed referral for diagnosis and treatment. Figure 6.1 presents the infrastructure and workflow of the screening information system.

6.2.1 Pre-screening Phase

The pre-screening phase makes use of the information from claimed data, cancer registry data, death registry data, and household registry to filter and identify the eligible population to be invited.

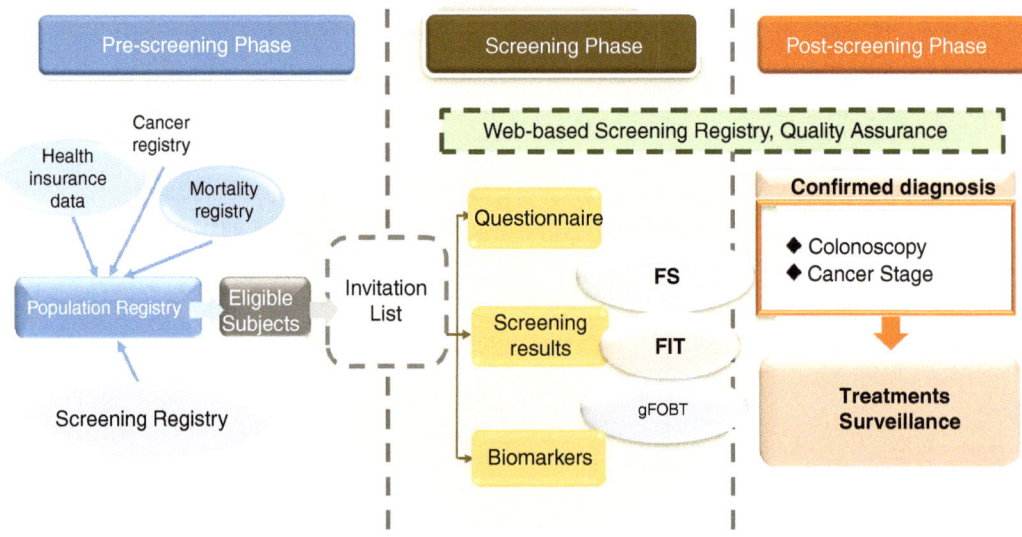

Fig. 6.1 Infrastructure and workflow of a screening information system

6.2.2 Screening Phase

The screening phase begins with registration. The output of the pre-screening phase is exactly the input of the screening phase. During the screening phase, the results of the collected information, including questionnaires, the results of screening results (i.e., FIT kit brand, FIT positivity, and quantitative measurements of FIT) are recorded and stored with a web-based system. Additional information such as the results of biomarkers can also be collected using the platform of multiple disease screening program. This information facilitates the monitoring of screening process indicators such as the uptake of screening (or participation rate) and positivity rate.

6.2.3 Post-screening Phase

In the post-screening phase, attendees with positive screening tests are provided with diagnostic examinations such as colonoscopy and subsequent clinical management if a neoplasm is detected. The findings of diagnostic examination,

histology of detected neoplasm, stage of screen-detected CRCs, and the provision of treatment, can be derived via integrated information system linking the screening database, cancer registry, and other external databases together. Based on these results, the compliance rate of colonoscopy (or diagnostic examination rate) and cancer (or neoplasm) detection rate can be evaluated. These process indicators are the cardinal elements for quality assurance in the organized screening program. Figure 6.2 shows the user interface of the standardized colonoscopy reporting format in the picture archiving and communication system (PACS) system that is currently used in Taiwanese program.

Based on the flow of CRC screening and the collected multiple source data, the stepwise evaluation of the screening program includes the immediate indicator such as positivity rate, colonoscopy rate, positive predictive value and detection rate, the early outcome of stage shifting, the intermediate outcome of interval cancer rate, and the long-term outcome of mortality or incidence reduction. The information system integrating the digitalized data from health care providers and public health administrators into a central database also make it

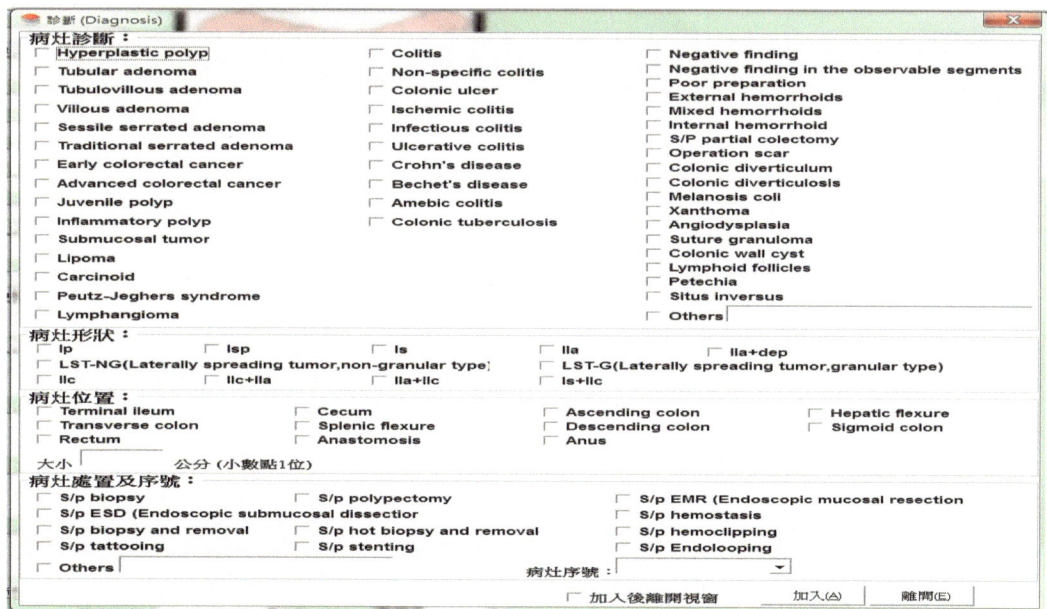

Fig. 6.2 Uniform Colonoscopy Report Format that currently used in Taiwanese program (*Courtesy of professor Han-Mo Chiu of National Taiwan University Hospital*)

possible to provide the real-time monitoring and feedback on the quality issues such as bowel preparation, cecal intubation rate, and adenoma detection rate. By the current information technology, the information system can be designed to reach the parallel linkage within the health care systems and the horizontal linkage across the health care organizations.

Data visualization combines data analysis methods with interactive visualization to enable comprehensive data exploration. Presenting information is a key challenge that needs to be met in order for decision makers to be able to properly analyze screening data. For example, the bubble chart for each screening setting shows a comparison that allows for each differentiation of the adenoma detection rate between screening settings by bubble sizes (the volume of colonoscopy). The average adenoma detection rate at the national level could be reported as a reference for those who have a lower adenoma detection rate to improve the quality of colonoscopy. Similarly, the quality issues about the implementation of CRC programs including short- and long-term outcomes could be monitored by the designed information system. For example, the proportion of early-stage CRC accounts for the screen- and clinical-detected cancers as an early indicator for short-term evaluation.

6.3 Fundamental Indicators and Databases for Supporting Implementation and Evaluation of CRC Screening

While implementing the organized population-based screening, some essential indicators and databases are required to technically support the screening procedure and a broad range of perspectives in the pre-screening, screening, and post-screening phases during the processes of screening (Chiu et al. 2006). The essential indicators and relevant databases in pre-screening, screening, and post-screening phases present in Fig. 6.3.

6.3.1 Pre-screening Phase

The following three databases should be prepared before launching CRC service screening:

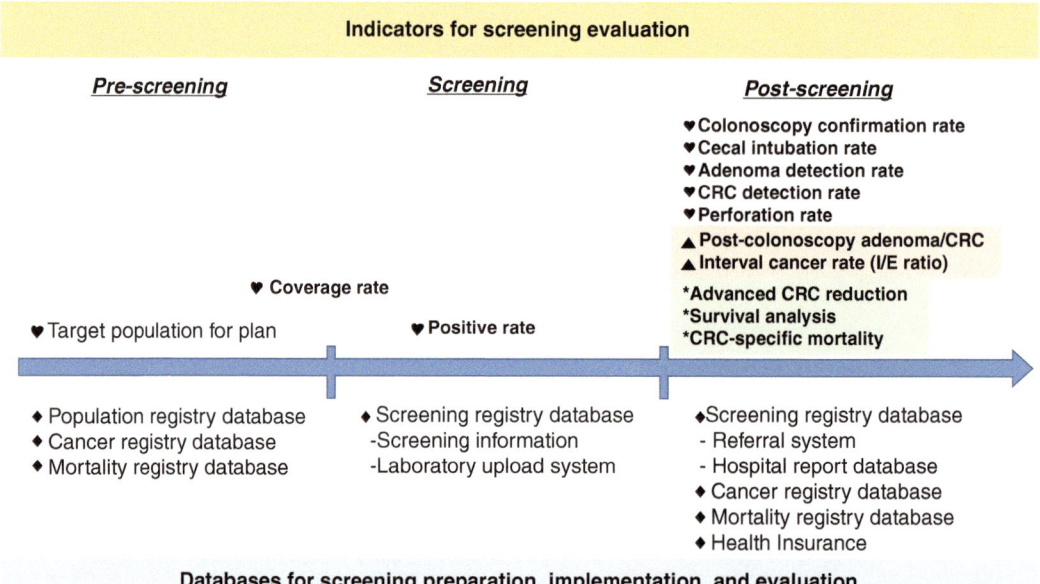

Fig. 6.3 The essential indicators and databases in different phases of organized CRC screening program

1. Population Household Registry Data

    The population registry data is one of the fundamental elements for screening programs. The main purposes of using population registry data are: (1) to quantify the eligible targeted population based on available budgets or medical resources at the initial stage; (2) to invite the targeted population for colorectal cancer screening.

2. Mortality (death) Registry Data

    Through the linkage process, subjects ascertained as death through mortality registry are excluded from invitation list. The death registry has good agreement (Kappa = 0.97) for malignant neoplasms (Lu et al. 2000). The mortality analysis based on mortality registry can be applied to evaluating the effectiveness of colorectal cancer screening program.

3. Cancer Registry Data

    The population registry data is another fundamental element for screening programs. The cancer registry is used to determine whether the subject has been diagnosed as colorectal cancer before screening. Subjects with previously certain diagnosed colorectal cancer are not invited to attend screening for colorectal cancer. The cancer registry is a nationwide program with a high coverage rate of 97% and a high accuracy rate of 99% (Chiang et al. 2015).

6.3.2 Screening Phase

Information on personal information, screening findings, necessary referrals, and confirmatory examinations should be collected and formed as the screening registry database in the screening phase. Taking the FIT screening as an example, the information for personal characteristics (e.g., living area, gender, and age), screening information (such as return date of test, uptake date, brand, and screening settings), and screening finding (test result and fecal hemoglobin concentration) should be collected. Some indicators for quality control in the screening phase should be monitored as well, such as the screening rate or test performance. The screening rate can be eval-

uated by using both the population registry and the screening registry databases (Chiu et al. 2015). The test performance, such as interval cancer, can be obtained by the linkage of screening registry data with cancer registry data. Moreover, for subjects with positive findings, the indicators for quality management in referral process not only focus on the compliance of confirmatory colonoscopy but also the waiting time of colonoscopy (Jen et al. 2018). The quality of the screening program could be improved by regular monitoring. In this phase, the major indicators and databases are elaborated as follows.

1. Compliance, Waiting time, and Quality Control of Colonoscopy

    For subjects who need to undergo colonoscopy, the results from colonoscopy should be recorded. The compliance of colonoscopy is one of the quality indicators for CRC screening programs. The compliance rate of receiving colonoscopy could be adjusted with test positive with referrals. The waiting time for colonoscopy confirmation is defined by the duration between the date of FIT examination and the date of colonoscopy completion. The longer waiting time is, the more likely to have interval cancer. As per the guideline for CRC screening, those who are FIT positive cases should be referred to clinics/hospitals for colonoscopy confirmation within a duration of lesser than three months. Using the screening registry database, the duration for confirmation can be calculated individually to monitor the duration of waiting time, which might be affected by clinical workforce capacity, health awareness, and cultural reasons (Cheng et al. 2018).

    Other indicators for colonoscopy procedures such as the bowel cleaning status, colonoscopy reach deep, and pathology reports for quality control of colonoscopy in referral system. The essential indicators in post-screening phase are elaborated as follows:

(a) Colonoscopy Rate

$$= \frac{\text{completed colonocsopy confirmation}}{\text{Total FIT positive cases}}$$

(b) Cecal Intubation Rate

$$= \frac{\text{colonoscopy reaching cecal location}}{\text{completed colonoscopy confirmation cases}}$$

(c) Adenoma Detection Rate

$$= \frac{\text{colonoscopy finding with adenoma(s)}}{\text{completed colonoscopy confirmation cases}}$$

(d) Advanced Adenoma Detection Rate

$$= \frac{\text{colonoscopy finding with advanced adenoma(s)}}{\text{completed colonoscopy confirmation cases}}$$

(e) CRC Detection Rate

$$\text{CRC detection rate} = \frac{\text{colonoscopy finding with CRC}}{\text{completed colonoscopy confirmation cases}}$$

2. Early Indicator for Evaluation of Advanced Stage CRC Reduction

Early detection of CRC is the first goal of colorectal cancer screening. Stage shifting of CRC from late toward early stages (comparing subjects who did with those who did not participate in screening) can be used as a short-term or early indicator of a screening program. First, the stage information is either collecting from hospitals or obtaining from cancer registry data. Comparing the stage distribution before and after implementation of screening program, or comparison of the stage distribution of CRC detected by different detection modes (screening-detected CRC and those diagnosed after symptom) as described in Chap. 2 are two commonly used approaches (Zorzi and Fedeli 2015; Chiu et al. 2015).

3. Test and Colonoscopy Interval Cancers

As mentioned in Chap. 2 regarding the definition of interval cancers, symptomatic CRCs diagnosed after negative FIT and before the next round of screening are defined as FIT interval cancer whereas the symptomatic CRCs diagnosed before the subsequent colonoscopy at recommended surveillance interval in subjects without the diagnosis of CRC at baseline colonoscopy are defined as colonoscopy interval cancers (Sanduleanu et al. 2015). They are usually identified through a linkage of screening database with the cancer registry. The interval cancer can be considered as a mid-term indicator for the performance of screening. In FIT screening program, the performance of FIT can be improved by the better use of fecal hemoglobin concentration (FHbC), the quantitative measurement of fecal hemoglobin level in FIT (Chen et al. 2011, 2013; Yen et al. 2014). It can be used to stratify the population into different risk groups and tailor them with different inter-screening intervals. Subjects with higher FHbC can be considered as higher risk population and a shorter inter-screening interval can be assigned and those with lower FHbC can be offered next round of FIT with longer intervals. For those with extremely high FHbC, the subsequent risk of CRC is very high and direct use of colonoscopy rather than FIT could be considered for the next round of screening. Both false negative and false positive cases could be reduced by such a stool-based personalized screening strategy (Chen et al. 2018). Even after colonoscopy, FHbC can also play a major role in stratifying subjects into different risk groups, according to our previous study (Chiu et al. 2017).

6.3.3 Post-screening Phase

1. Surveillance After Removal of Colorectal Adenomatous Polyps

Surveillance after removal of adenoma provides additional protection against incident CRC caused by missed or newly developed neoplasms. The appropriate surveillance after adenoma removal should be carried out according to the recommended interval recommended by major guidelines (Hassan et al. 2013; Gupta et al. 2020). The patient demographics, baseline colonoscopic findings, the presence of comorbidity, the presence of other risk factors, timing, and results for surveillance examination should be collected in order to monitor the appropriateness of surveillance procedures and relevant risk factors of colonoscopy interval cancers. Surveillance of adenoma and advanced adenoma can be also implemented by the stratification of f-Hb concentration.

2. Evaluation of Effectiveness of CRC Screening

The primary long-term outcome of CRC screening is mainly based on mortality reduction from CRC (Chiu et al. 2015; Lee et al. 2018). The long-term outcome in advanced CRC by early detection should further be evaluated. The incidence reduction by screening program would be also expected because of the removal of adenomatous polyps.

3. Economic Evaluation

Cost-effectiveness analysis (CEA), cost-utility analysis (CUA), and cost-benefit analysis (CBA) under the context of economic evaluation have been recognized as one of the essential domains of evidence-based medicine. The comprehensive databases enable collection of data regarding costs or medical expenditures during the process of screening or treatment as well as the evidence on effectiveness of screening to do economic evaluation as described in Chap. 10.

4. Evaluation of Personalized Screening for CRC

In order to render population-based organized service screening effective and cost-effective, personalized screening strategy has been recommended in recent years by making use of demographic features, genetic determinants, environmental risk factors, and available biomarkers to stratify the targeted population into different risk groups. In recent years, f-Hb concentration derived from FIT has been strongly recommended as a good predictor for individualized risk profiles for CRC. Screening policies such as age to begin with screen, inter-screening interval, and the use of alternative advanced screening tools can be expediently applied to a constellation of subgroups. Health information on all these aspects pertaining to individual risk profiles had better be well collected before the development of personalized strategies for CRC.

Health information system supporting population-based organized service screening for CRC can help health professionals to improve the quality assurance and to evaluate the screening program. It is determined by the infrastructure of the screening program, availability and comprehensiveness of screening data, and the sophisticated and precise data analysis with adjustment for potential biases. The infrastructure of the screening process includes three phases: pre-screening, screening, and post-screening phase. A centralized integrated database linking various kinds of databases together from pre-screening phase makes contribution to planning population-based organized service screening. Data on the key performance index collected in screening phase includes the screening rate, positive rate, referral rate, positive predictive rate, detection rate, and interval cancer rate. Data collected from post-screening phase include surveillance of adenoma, effectiveness and cost-effectiveness evaluation, and the personalized strategies for colorectal cancer screening.

Building up a systematic health information system for population-based organized service screening is of importance to develop evidence-based screening policy beyond randomized controlled trial and may facilitate personalized strategy for CRC screening.

References

Chen LS, Yen AM, Chiu SY, Liao CS, Chen HH. Baseline faecal occult blood concentration as a predictor of incident colorectal neoplasia: longitudinal follow-up of a Taiwanese population-based colorectal cancer screening cohort. Lancet Oncol. 2011;12(6):551–8.

Chen LS, Yen AM, Fraser CG, Chiu SY, Fann JC, Wang PE, Lin SC, Liao CS, Lee YC, Chiu HM, Chen

HH. Impact of faecal haemoglobin concentration on colorectal cancer mortality and all-cause death. BMJ Open. 2013;3(11):e003740.

Chen SL, Hsu CY, Yen AM, Young GP, Chiu SY, Fann JC, Lee YC, Chiu HM, Chiou ST, Chen HH. Demand for colonoscopy in colorectal Cancer screening using a quantitative fecal immunochemical test and age/sex-specific thresholds for test positivity. Cancer Epidemiol Biomark Prev. 2018 Jun;27(6):704–9.

Cheng SY, Li MC, Chia SL, Huang KC, Chiu TY, Chan DC, Chiu HM. Factors affecting compliance with confirmatory colonoscopy after a positive fecal immunochemical test in a national colorectal screening program. Cancer. 2018;124(5):907–15.

Chiang CJ, You SL, Chen CJ, Yang YW, Lo WC, Lai MS. Quality assessment and improvement of nationwide cancer registration system in Taiwan: a review. Jpn J Clin Oncol. 2015;45(3):291–6.

Chiu YH, Chen LS, Chan CC, Liou DM, Wu SC, Kuo HS, Chang HJ, Chen TH. Health information system for community-based multiple screening in Keelung, Taiwan (Keelung community-based integrated screening no. 3). Int J Med Inform. 2006;75(5):369–83.

Chiu HM, Chen SL, Yen AM, Chiu SY, Fann JC, Lee YC, Pan SL, Wu MS, Liao CS, Chen HH, Koong SL, Chiou ST. Effectiveness of fecal immunochemical testing in reducing colorectal cancer mortality from the one million Taiwanese screening program. Cancer. 2015;121(18):3221–9.

Chiu SY, Chuang SL, Chen SL, Yen AM, Fann JC, Chang DC, Lee YC, Wu MS, Chou CK, Hsu WF, Chiou ST, Chiu HM. Faecal haemoglobin concentration influences risk prediction of interval cancers resulting from inadequate colonoscopy quality: analysis of the Taiwanese Nationwide Colorectal Cancer Screening Program. Gut. 2017;66(2):293–300.

Gupta S, Lieberman D, Anderson JC, Burke CA, Dominitz JA, Kaltenbach T, Robertson DJ, Shaukat A, Syngal S, Rex DK. Recommendations for follow-up after colonoscopy and polypectomy: a consensus update by the US multi-society task force on colorectal Cancer. Gastroenterology. 2020;158(4):1131–53.

Hassan C, Quintero E, Dumonceau JM, et al. Post-polypectomy colonoscopy surveillance: European Society of Gastrointestinal Endoscopy (ESGE) guideline. Endoscopy. 2013;45(10):842–51.

Jen HH, Hsu CY, Chen SL, et al. Rolling-out screening volume affecting compliance rate and waiting time of FIT-based colonoscopy. J Clin Gastroenterol. 2018;52(9):821–7.

Lee YC, Hsu CY, Chen SL, Yen AM, Chiu SY, Fann JC, Chuang SL, Hsu WF, Chiang TH, Chiu HM, Wu MS, Chen HH. Effects of screening and universal healthcare on long-term colorectal cancer mortality. Int J Epidemiol. 2018 Sep 3;48:538. https://doi.org/10.1093/ije/dyy182.

Lu TH, Lee MC, Chou MC. Accuracy of cause-of-death coding in Taiwan: types of miscoding and effects on mortality statistics. Int J Epidemiol. 2000;29(2):336–43.

Sanduleanu S, le Clercq CM, Dekker E, et al. Definition and taxonomy of interval colorectal cancers: a proposal for standardising nomenclature. Gut. 2015;64(8):1257–67.

Yen AM, Chen SL, Chiu SY, Fann JC, Wang PE, Lin SC, Chen YD, Liao CS, Yeh YP, Lee YC, Chiu HM, Chen HH. A new insight into fecal hemoglobin concentration-dependent predictor for colorectal neoplasia. Int J Cancer. 2014 Sep 1;135(5):1203–12.

Zorzi M, Fedeli U. Early effect of screening programmes on incidence and mortality rates of colorectal cancer. Gut. 2015;64(6):1007.

Quality Assurance in Colorectal Cancer Screening Program

7

Han-Mo Chiu

Abstract

In an organized screening, quality assurance by setting targets to be met and continuous monitoring of key indicators using the relevant data collected within a program is its major difference from opportunistic screening. Those key indicators are frequently monitored and evaluated by the screening organizer to ensure that screening is well delivered and conducted. In organized colorectal cancer (CRC) screening program, screening test uptake, diagnostic examination compliance, screening test performance, and diagnostic examinations are closely associated with the effectiveness in preventing CRC and CRC death. Though CRC incidence or mortality is the most robust outcome to measure the performance of a screening program, it usually takes a long time to observe. Several quality metrics were developed, validated, and have been demonstrated to be associated with important outcomes (i.e., CRC incidence or mortality), it is of utmost importance to implement quality assurance mechanism in a pro-

H.-M. Chiu (✉)
Department of Internal Medicine, National Taiwan University Hospital, Taipei, Taiwan

Department of Internal Medicine, College of Medicine, National Taiwan University, Taipei, Taiwan
e-mail: hanmochiu@ntu.edu.tw

gram. In this chapter, those important quality indicators will be introduced and discussed.

Keywords

Colorectal Cancer (CRC) · Quality · Interval Cancer (IC) · Adenoma Detection Rate (ADR) · Fecal Immunochemical Test (FIT)

7.1 Overview

Colorectal cancer (CRC) screening involves multiple steps, starting from engaging people to go for noninvasive screening test [in most of the case guaiac fecal occult blood test (gFOBT) or fecal immunochemical test (FIT)], referral of subjects with positive screening tests to diagnostic examination (colonoscopy) to offering treatment for screening-detected neoplasm and risk-stratified regular surveillance after treatment. Each step is associated with several quality issues and the impact of quality on CRC screening program is remarkable (Fig. 7.1). This is rather easy to understand, because poor quality of screening may lead to undetected adenoma and early-stage cancer, leading to the development or progression of cancer that can only be diagnosed at a more advanced stage or when become symptomatic, which require more expense to treat but with more unfavorable survival. Quality assurance of

© Springer Nature Singapore Pte Ltd. 2021
H.-M. Chiu, H.-H. Chen (eds.), *Colorectal Cancer Screening*,
https://doi.org/10.1007/978-981-15-7482-5_7

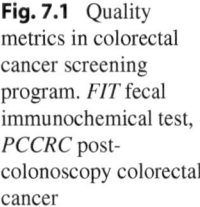

Fig. 7.1 Quality metrics in colorectal cancer screening program. *FIT* fecal immunochemical test, *PCCRC* post-colonoscopy colorectal cancer

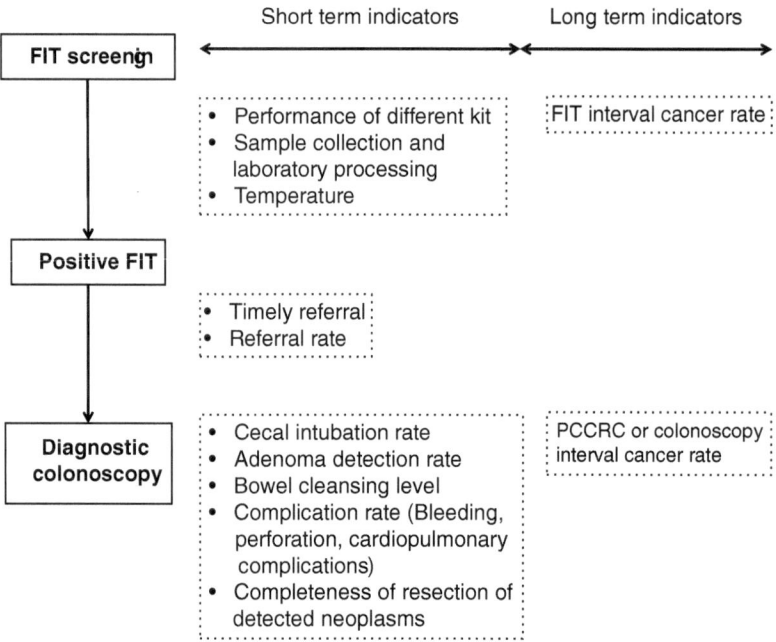

CRC screening program is multifaceted, ranging from the quality of FIT, colonoscopy quality represented by adenoma detection rate (ADR), cecal intubation rate (CIR), completeness of the treatment of detected neoplasms, and colonoscopy-related complication. Only when the quality of each step is secured then we can achieve higher effectiveness and cost-effectiveness of the entire screening program.

Quality assurance is more easily to be implemented in the organized screening program than in the opportunistic program because it provides screening service within a well-defined population and setting thereby enables better control of quality and safety during a complex screening process, timely subsequent management of screening-detected lesions, and evaluation of the outcome after certain quality assurance interventions.

Previous studies from Canada revealed that the risk of post-colonoscopy CRC was higher if polypectomy rate or complete rate of colonoscopy was low, or colonoscopy was performed by non-gastroenterologist, as those procedures are related with lower ADR and CIR (Singh et al. 2010a, b; Baxter et al. 2011). Several modeling studies also demonstrated that if screening colonoscopy was performed with insufficient quality

(represented by non-gastroenterologist performed colonoscopy or colonoscopy with low ADR) then there was less number of CRC averted, with more advanced stage CRC and CRC death, leading to less survival, more treatment-related cost and lower cost-effectiveness of screening (Hassan et al. 2012a; Meester et al. 2015) (Table 7.1).

7.2 Fecal Immunochemical Test-Related Quality Issues

FIT, like guaiac fecal occult blood test (gFOBT), enables the selection of subjects at higher likelihood of having invasive cancer or advanced adenoma. An accumulating body of evidence demonstrated that FIT outperforms guaiac FOBT and it is nowadays the most popular primary screening test worldwide. A meta-analysis of randomized controlled trials comparing gFOBT and FIT found that FIT detects more than twice as many CRCs and advanced adenomas (RR: 2.28, 95% CI = 1.68–3.10) (Hassan et al. 2012b). In cohort studies comparing gFOBT and FIT where all patients had colonoscopy, FIT also detected approximately twice as many CRCs and advanced adenomas than gFOBT and fewer colonoscopies

Table 7.1 Various major colorectal cancer screening quality indicators with their advantages and disadvantages

Indicators	Advantages	Disadvantages
Population level		
CRC mortality or incidence rate	Most robust outcome indicators and directly reflects screening effectiveness	• Requires 5–10 years to observe. • Difficult to use for immediate feedback. • Require a large sample size to calculate. • Require a comprehensive death or cancer registry covering the entire screening population.

Interval cancer (IC) rate	• Surrogate of program sensitivity.
	• Definition:
	  - *FIT IC*: CRC that becomes symptomatic and diagnosed after a negative FIT and before next round of FIT screening (Sanduleanu et al. 2015).
	  - *Colonoscopy IC*: CRC that becomes symptomatic and diagnosed after colonoscopy within the recommended surveillance interval (Sanduleanu et al. 2015).
		• Require a cancer registry covering the entire screening population.
		• Rather complicated in calculation.
		• Its magnitude may vary along with the kit that used, the screening interval or the cutoff used to define positivity, therefore, benchmark threshold is difficult to set (FIT interval cancer).
		• Difficult to verify and sometimes require a review of medical records (colonoscopy IC).

Unit/individual level		
Colonoscopy rate (after a positive screening test such as FIT or gFOBT)	• May directly affect screening effectiveness (Rabeneck et al. 2010; Lee et al. 2017). • Easy to calculate. • Benchmark threshold: 80% (Robertson et al. 2017).	• None.

Adenoma detection rate	• Demonstrated to be associated with IC, advanced stage CRC, or CRC death.
	• Can be verified with pathology.
	• Population level is rather simple and clear.
	• Benchmark threshold:
	  - Colonoscopy-based screening: Male: 30%, female: 20% (Rex et al. 2015).
	  - FIT-based screening: 30–40% (Robertson et al. 2017; Jover et al. 2012; Bronzwaer et al. 2019).
		• Benchmark threshold may vary along with an ethnic group, population demographics (age, gender, or risk factors such as smoking and obesity). and setting (colonoscopy screening vs. FIT screening).
		• Its applicability and benchmark level for surveillance colonoscopy is unclear.
		• May not be associated with the detection of SSA/P.
		• "One-and-done" phenomenon (resect one adenoma and ignore other co-existent adenomas) exists.

Cecal intubation rate	• Demonstrated to be associated with PCCRC or colonoscopy IC. (Baxter et al. 2011, Chiu et al. 2017) • Benchmark threshold: 95% (Rex et al. 2015; Jover et al. 2012; Bronzwaer et al. 2019; Kaminski et al. 2017a).	• Rely on self-reporting without objective verification process thus misreporting may exist. • Still debating on its definition.
Bowel cleansing level	• Validated and easy to use scoring system exits (i.e. BBPS). • Closely associated with neoplasm detection rate (Harewood et al. 2003).	• No study relates it with CRC incidence. • May surrogate to ADR .
Colonoscopy related complication rate	• Relevant to the safety issue of CRC screening. • Perforation: <1/1000 (Jover et al. 2012; Kaminski et al. 2017a; Chilton et al. 2011). • Severe bleeding: <1/100 (Chilton et al. 2011).	• Surveillance system is needed. • Definition may vary (bleeding). • Misreporting may exist.

were required to detect one advanced lesion (Brenner and Tao 2013; Park et al. 2010; Graser et al. 2009).

Its single test sensitivity in detecting CRC is not perfect, being reported to be 79% in a meta-analysis, and is usually recommended to undergo in one- or two-year intervals (Robertson et al. 2017; Lee et al. 2014). The performances of different FIT kits have been introduced and compared in Chap. 5.

Several issues are important regarding FIT testing including pre-laboratory processes, laboratory organization, analytical methods, and post-laboratory processes (Kelly et al. 2017). Each step is associated with the accuracy of FIT and may affect the screening outcomes. False-negative FIT may lead to symptomatic CRC that occurs during the inter-screening interval (FIT interval cancer) and affect the effectiveness of the screening program. False-positive tests may lead to increased demand for colonoscopy hence increase the cost and compromise the efficiency of the screening. Some studies have compared the performance of different FIT kits, including qualitative and quantitative ones, and revealed that they may be largely different in terms of detecting CRC and advanced adenoma, stability in high temperature, the amount of stool samples taken using the spatula (Park et al. 2012). In some programs, more than one FIT kits or mixed quantitative or qualitative FIT kits are used within the same program but without the mechanism of regular evaluation and comparison of their performance at a short or long time span. Chiang et al. compared the two FIT kits that were used in Taiwanese program and demonstrated that the risk of incident CRC within 2 years after negative FITs (FIT interval cancer) using those two brands of quantitative FITs, even with the same cutoff hemoglobin concentration, was significantly different, highlighting the importance of population-level analysis to verify the credibility of quantitative laboratory findings (Chiang et al. 2014). In a recent study from the Korean CRC screening program, in which both quantitative and qualitative FITs were used, revealed that interval cancer risk was significantly higher in the qualitative FIT group (aOR 1.31, 95% CI

1.12–1.52). Moreover, interval cancer risk was significantly higher in subjects who received FIT screening in summer season (aOR 1.16, 95% CI 1.07–1.27) (Cha et al. 2018).

7.3 Colonoscopy-Related Quality Issues

Colonoscopy is considered as the most complicated step in the whole CRC screening process, as it requires dietary restriction and bowel preparation prior to the procedure and the examination itself is invasive and associated with the risk of complication. It is the common pathway of all screening tests and considered as the gold-standard diagnostic exam after positive non-invasive screening tests (e.g., gFOBT, FIT, or blood markers). It plays a pivotal role to detect and treat (either colonoscopic polypectomy or referral for surgical resection) neoplasms in a screening program. Securing its quality is of utmost importance for maximizing its effectiveness in preventing CRC. Measuring outcomes like interval CRC rate or PCCRC rate would be theoretically the most robust way to reflect the effectiveness of colonoscopy in preventing CRC. Using it as a quality indicator, however, has disadvantages including that it requires a very long period of time to observe the outcome (interval cancer or PCCRC) therefore is unsuitable to sue for timely feedback to the individual operator or endoscopic unit, and it also requires a huge number of procedures and a large number of cancer cases to obtain precise estimations, which also affects its feasibility to use (Rutter et al. 2018). Moreover, there is wide variation in the colonoscopy IC or PCCRC rate (Robertson et al. 2014; Chiu et al. 2017). Some of this may derive from different study design—especially data origin, exclusion criteria, and population studied (screening setting: colonoscopy- or FIT-based screening), and from method of calculation that used, therefore, it is difficult to determine a benchmark threshold for colonoscopy IC or PCCRC (Robertson et al. 2014). Nevertheless, screening organizer still should monitor the magnitude of interval CRC within the program to identify outliers, because interval cancer rate actually reflects the performance of a screening program (program sensitivity) and many factors associated with colonoscopy IC or PCCRC are operator or system factors that can be ameliorated via quality assurance interventions. Currently, there is a consensus on the definition of PCCRC and colonoscopy IC by an international expert panel (Sanduleanu et al. 2015; Rutter et al. 2018).

7.3.1 Timely Referral (In FIT Program)

FIT positivity represents a high-risk condition and subjects with positive FIT have 20–30 times higher risk of CRC compared with the general population. If subjects are not compliant with diagnostic colonoscopy after positive FIT then the risk of dying from CRC was 64% higher compared with those who were compliant according to the data from the Taiwanese program (Lee et al. 2017). The diagnostic colonoscopy rate after FIT varies across programs, with 82.8% in the Netherlands, 88.9% in the United Kingdom, 68.1% in Japan, 46.6% in Korea, and 80% in Taiwan (Lee et al. 2017; Lo et al. 2015; RIVM Dutch Colorectal Cancer Screening Programme 2018, Ministry of Helath. Labour, and Welfare of Japanese government. 2016; Chiu et al. 2015; Rim et al. 2017). Several barriers exist for non-compliance to colonoscopy in FIT screening program, and physician's recommendation has been reported to play the most important role (Cheng et al. 2018). In UK NHS bowel screening program and Irish National Cancer Screening service, the standard of colonoscopy rate after positive FOBT was set at 85% (Kelly et al. 2017; Chilton 2011). The US Multi-Society Task Force on Colorectal Cancer recommend colonoscopy completion rate for those with a positive FIT of 80% or greater (Robertson et al. 2017).

Timely colonoscopy is also important because prolonged waiting time may increase the risk of malignant transformation from advanced adenoma to invasive cancer or progression of early-stage CRC to advanced stage ones. A study from the United States revealed that if the time from positive FIT to colonoscopy was 10–12 months then the risks of CRC and advanced stage CRC were significantly higher with OR of 1.48 [95% CI, 1.05–2.08] and 1.97 [95% CI, 1.14–3.42], respectively. If the time was even longer than 12 months then OR was 2.25 [95% CI, 1.89–2.68] for CRC and 3.22 [95% CI, 2.44–4.25] for advanced stage CRC (Corley et al. 2017). Similar study from Taiwanese program also revealed that every one-month delay of diagnostic colonoscopy resulted in 1% increased risk of CRC and 4% increased risk of advanced-stage CRC (Lee et al. 2019).

7.3.2 Bowel Preparation

Adequate bowel preparation is essential to ensure safe, efficient, and comprehensive colonoscopy examination in terms of higher both cecal intubation and adenoma detection rates (Harewood et al. 2003; Bernstein et al. 2005; Jaruvongvanich et al. 2018). Studies have shown that high-risk neoplasm might have missed if bowel preparation was inadequate (Chokshi et al. 2012; Lebwohl et al. 2011). To achieve better bowel preparation, based on the abundant body of evidence, major guidelines recommend same-day preparation or split-dose preparation being the preferred way of conducting bowel preparation (ASGE Standards of Practice Committee 2015; Johnson et al. 2014; Hassan et al. 2019; Clark et al. 2014; Chiu et al. 2006; Radaelli et al. 2017; Bucci et al. 2014; Martel et al. 2015). Regarding the regimen for bowel preparation, most of the guidelines recommend Polyethylene Glycol Electrolyte lavage solution (PEG-ELS) as the first-line regimen. Other regimens, such as oral sulfate solution and sodium picosulfate/magnesium citrate can also be used for bowel preparation with similar cleansing effect as PEG-ELS (Regev et al. 1998; Manes et al. 2013). Sodium phosphate solution, though effective and well-tolerated, is no more recommended as the first-line agent for bowel preparation for colonoscopy because of the rare occurrence of phosphate nephropathy (Markowitz et al. 2005; Choi et al. 2014).

Table 7.2 Bowel preparation scales that used in different programs (Bronzwaer et al. 2019; Kelly et al. 2017; Chilton et al. 2011; Colonoscopy quality standards and quality metrics in Taiwan)

Program	Benchmark threshold	Scale
Netherlands	BBPS of 6 or higher in at least 90% of colonoscopies	Boston bowel preparation scale (BBPS)
Ireland	Bowel preparation described as Excellent or adequate: >90%	Aronchick scale
Taiwan	Adequate preparation (excellent, good, and fair) >90%	Aronchick scale
UK	Bowel preparation of sufficient diagnostic quality to not warrant repeat or alternative test: >90%	Aronchick scale

There are several scoring systems for bowel preparation, including Aronchick, Boston, and Ottawa Bowel Preparation Scales (Parmar et al. 2016). Among them, the Boston Bowel Preparation Scale is the most thoroughly validated scale and is recommended to use in a clinical setting. Different scales were used in individual programs, such as Aronchick scale in UK, Irish, and Taiwanese programs and Boston scale in Dutch Colorectal Cancer Screening Program (Rees et al. 2016; Bronzwaer et al. 2019; Kelly et al. 2017; Colonoscopy quality standards and quality metrics in Taiwan). Benchmark threshold for bowel preparation adequacy was also set in several programs (Table 7.2).

7.3.3 Cecal Intubation Rate or Complete Colonoscopy Rate

A complete examination of the entire colon is a fundamental objective of colonoscopy and a key performance indicator. Several population-based studies have demonstrated that completeness of colonoscopy was associated with the risk of PCCRC or colonoscopy interval cancers (Baxter et al. 2011; Chiu et al. 2017; Hilsden et al. 2015). Baxter et al. further demonstrated that incomplete colonoscopy was not only associated with a

higher risk of incident cancers at proximal colon but also distal colon (Baxter et al. 2011). This is not difficult to understand, because endoscopists who have lower rate of complete colonoscopy may be less skillful not only for scope insertion but also for neoplasm detection. Currently, cecal intubation is generally self-reported, either by endoscopists or nursing staffs, lacking formal verification process. Nevertheless, major guidelines and screening programs have set a standard of 90 or 95% cecal intubation rate and photographic evidence of either the ICV or the appendix orifice must be archived to support completion colonoscopy (Rex et al. 2015; Bronzwaer et al. 2019; Kaminski et al. 2017a; Kelly et al. 2017; Chilton et al. 2011; Colonoscopy quality standards and quality metrics in Taiwan; Australian Institute of Health and Welfare. 2014).

7.3.4 Adenoma Detection Rate

An endoscopist's adenoma detection rate (ADR) is the proportion of individuals undergoing a complete screening colonoscopy who have one or more adenomas detected. It is widely used as the benchmark quality measure for colonoscopy. ADR of 30% is the benchmark threshold proposed by USMSTF (35% for men and 25% for women) (check) and 25% by ESGE (Rex et al. 2015; Kaminski et al. 2017a). The ADR in FIT screening program, however, should theoretically be higher than that in the primary screening colonoscopy setting because FIT positive subjects represent a high-risk population having higher likelihood of neoplasm. The true adenoma burden in FIT positive subjects could vary based on factors such as the threshold used to define a positive FIT, individual screening program may need to calculate its own benchmarks using local data (Hilsden et al. 2016). A recent Asia-Pacific multi-country study involving 2901 subjects who received primary screening colonoscopy and 2485 subjects who received diagnostic colonoscopy due to positive FIT revealed that ADR (53.6% vs. 37.5%; odds ratio [OR], 1.93; $P < 0.001$) and advanced adenoma detection rate (29.9% vs. 4.9%; OR, 8.2; $P < 0.001$) were both significantly higher in colonoscopy for FIT positive subjects than the corresponding values for primary screening colonoscopy indicating that benchmark threshold of ADR for FIT positive subjects should be set at higher level (Wong et al. 2019).

There are several cohort studies demonstrating the close association of ADR with subsequent risk of post-colonoscopy CRC or colonoscopy interval cancers (Table 7.3). Kaminski et al. firstly demonstrated that ADR was inversely associated with the risk of interval CRC in the Polish program (Kaminski et al. 2017a). Baxter et al. demonstrated that low ADR is more likely associated with proximal PCCRC (Baxter et al. 2011). Corley et al. reported that not only was ADR inversely associated with the incidence of CRC, it was also inversely associated with the risk of advanced-stage CRC and CRC mortality, with each 1% increase in ADR associated with a 3% decreased risk of incident CRC and 5% decrease in CRC mortality. The only report from

the FIT-based screening program by Chiu et al. demonstrated that hospital-level ADR, together with cecal intubation rate and baseline colonoscopy findings, was associated with colonoscopy IC in FIT-based screening program (Chiu et al. 2017).

The benchmark threshold for ADR varies amongst different programs as it may be affected by adenoma prevalence in the population, the primary screening test (FIT or colonoscopy) that adopted in the program, and biological factors such as gender and age. Traditionally, the proportion of subjects with at least one neoplastic lesion among all subjects that received colonoscopy was the standard way to define ADR. It is, however, prone to be gamed and there is concern that endoscopists may focus on finding an adenoma, and once they have done so their attention may wane knowing they already earned credit toward the ADR leading to missed neoplasia (so-called "one and done" phenomenon: after identifying 1

Table 7.3 Studies demonstrating the association between ADR and incident CRC after colonoscopy

Author	Study population	Association of ADR and interval CRC risk
Kaminski et al. (2010)	Polish national CRC screening program, 45,026 subjects, 186 endoscopists	ADR: ≥0.20: Reference 0.15–0.199: HR = 10.94 (1.37–87.01) 0.11–0.149: HR = 10.75 (1.36–85.06) <0.11: HR = 12.50 (1.51–103.43)
Baxter et al. (2011)	34,312 individuals diagnosed with CRC, 2000–2005, Ontario cancer registry	ADR: Proximal CRC/distal CRC <0.1: Reference 0.1–0.14: 1.11 (0.81–1.53)/0.99 (0.73–1.35) 0.15–0.19: 0.75 (0.54–1.04)/0.78 (0.57–1.06) 0.20–0.24: 0.75 (0.52–1.07)/0.82 (0.58–1.16) 0.25–0.29: 0.52 (0.35–0.79)/0.87 (0.61–1.24) >30: 0.61 (0.42–0.89)/0.79 (0.54–1.14)
Cooper et al. (2012)	SEER, 57,839 patients aged 69 years that received colonoscopy during 1994–2005	Polypectomy rate: 0–0.24: Reference 0.24–0.33: OR = 0.84 (0.76–0.93) 0.33–0.43: OR = 0.80 (0.72–0.89) >0.43: OR = 0.70 (0.63–0.78)
Corley et al. (2014)	Kaiser Permanente northern California, 314,872 colonoscopies by 136 endoscopists during 1998–2010	ADR: 0.0735–0.1905: Reference 0.1906–0.2385: HR = 0.93 (0.70–1.23) 0.2386–0.2840: HR = 0.85 (0.68–1.06) 0.2841–0.3350: HR = 0.70 (0.54–0.91) 0.3351–0.5251: HR = 0.52 (0.39–0.69)
Chiu et al. (2017)	Taiwanese Nationwide CRC screening program, 29,969 subjects underwent complete colonoscopy after positive FIT during 2004–2009	ADR (hospital level) >0.3: Reference 0.30–0.15: HR = 1.57 (0.94–2.61) <0.15: HR = 3.09 (1.55–6.18)

adenomatous polyp, the endoscopist stops examining the remaining mucosa as carefully as before). Modified ADR metrics, such as APC (adenoma per colonoscopy), APP (adenoma per positive participant), ADR-plus may be considered as alternative quality measurements. This may be extraordinarily important in FIT-based screening because FIT positivity is associated with a higher likelihood of synchronous neoplasms and a more number of adenoma and one-and-done practice may obviously increase the risk of colonoscopy IC. Other similar metrics like polypectomy rate, proximal ADR, AADR (advanced adenoma detection rate), or SSADR (sessile serrated adenoma/polyp detection rate) are now under exploration (Aniwan et al. 2016; Ross et al. 2015; Wang et al. 2013; Gohel et al. 2014; Park et al. 2016; Greenspan et al. 2013).

ADR is ameliorable via educational intervention to endoscopists and sustained high ADR or improved from a low-to-high level of ADR was reported to be associated with lowered PCCRC or colonoscopy IC (Kaminski et al. 2017b).

7.3.5 Colonoscopy-Related Complications

Safety issues are an important consideration in a screening program. The most significant complication in CRC screening program is related to colonoscopy procedures, including colonoscopy per se, its associated procedures (biopsy or polypectomy) and conscious sedation. Colonoscopic adverse events are unusual but may be potentially life threatening. Major guidelines have addressed the importance of monitoring the colonoscopy-related complication but benchmark threshold is difficult to set, because the magnitude of complication rate may vary along with the definition of complication (perforation or severe bleeding, immediate, or delayed complications) and screening population.

Perforation is the most severe colonoscopy-related complication and it may result from direct mechanical trauma to the colonic wall during insertion, over-insufflation of the colon with resultant barotrauma to colonic wall, or as result of therapeutic procedures (hot biopsy or polypec-

tomy). Published rates of colonoscopic perforation and bleeding vary widely ranging from 0.07 to 0.4 per 1000 colonoscopies for perforations and between 0.8 and 2.4 per 1000 colonoscopies for post-colonoscopy bleeding (Rex et al. 2015; Kaminski et al. 2017a; Reumkens et al. 2016). ASGE guidelines define perforation rates of greater than 1/1000 in screening patients should initiate internal or external review to determine whether scope insertion or polypectomy practice is inappropriate whereas in ESGE guidelines there was no precise benchmark threshold for immediate complication rate but just set a minimum standard of $\leq 0.5\%$ for 7-day readmission rate (Rex et al. 2015). Some screening programs have set a threshold for colonoscopy related complication rates whereas in some programs the screening organizers request regular audit of severe complication, recording of immediate complication in the colonoscopy report, and regular morbidity or mortality conference to assess the causes of any complications and to discuss solutions to avoid them (Bronzwaer et al. 2019; Kelly et al. 2017).

Bleeding is another more common complication of colonoscopy. A variety of studies have reported polypectomy-associated bleeding rates of 0.3–6.1%. The risk of bleeding increases with the size of polyp and location, with some series reporting up to 10% bleeding rates for polyps larger than 2 cm located in the right colon (Reumkens et al. 2016; Parra-Blanco et al. 2000; Rosen et al. 1993). As the severity of bleeding may vary widely from self-limited minor bleeding to life-threatening hematochezia requiring hemostasis and admission, significant bleeding is usually defined as drop in hemoglobin of 2 g/dL or greater, bleeding that requires transfusion, hemostasis (either endoscopic or radiological), prolonged admission (>4 days) or surgery (Chilton 2011; Gavin et al. 2013) (Table 7.4). Most of the programs set a standard at <1 per 100 polypectomies. This benchmark threshold, however, may change over time because endoscopic resection of large colorectal adenoma becomes more popular which may increase the likelihood of polypectomy-associated bleeding but on the other hand the popularization of cold snare pol-

Table 7.4 Grade of post-colonoscopy/polypectomy bleeding as defined in the UK NHS Bowel Cancer Screening Program

Fetal	Death
Major	• Surgery. • Unplanned admission or prolongation of hospital stay for >10 nights. • Intensive care unit (ICU) admission >1 night.
Intermediate	• Hemoglobin drop ≥ 2 g/dL. • Transfusion. • Unplanned admission or prolongation of hospital stay for 4–10 nights. • ICU admission for 1 night. • Interventional procedure (endoscopic/radiological).
Minor	• Procedure aborted. • Unplanned post-procedure consultation. • Unplanned hospital admission or prolongation of. • Hospital stay for ≤ 3 nights.

Adapted from reference Rees et al. (2016)

ypectomy may reduce such risk. Moreover, FIT increases the likelihood of detecting advanced or synchronous adenoma, therefore the risk of polypectomy-associated bleeding may be higher in the FIT screening program and different standards may be required. Nevertheless, regular monitoring and audit of significant bleeding at either hospital or program level are mandatory.

As most of the post-polypectomy bleeding is caused by deep thermal injury of hot biopsy or hot snare polypectomy for small (<10 mm) polyps, ESGE guidelines suggest cold snare polypectomy for sessile polyps sized less than 10 mm because of its superiority in safety profile though direct evidence from a randomized controlled trial is still lacking (Ferlitsch et al. 2017).

7.3.6 Polyp Resection

Along with the advancement and popularity of endoscopic treatment techniques, the majority of adenoma detected by screening can be resected endoscopically. Routine referral of adenoma for surgery may expose the patients to the risk of operation or general anesthesia-related complications, prolonged admission, and increased cost. Even if the endoscopist is not confident in resecting the lesions endoscopically, he or she should refer the patient to other skillful specialists rather than referring directly to surgeons. In US guidelines, it was recommended that mucosally based pedunculated polyps and sessile Polyps less than 20 mm in size should not be sent for surgical

resection without an attempt at endoscopic resection or documentation of endoscopic inaccessibility (Rex et al. 2015). Incomplete resection of screening detected neoplasms was estimated to be responsible for 25% of PCCRC or colonoscopy interval cancers (Robertson et al. 2014; Chiu et al. 2017; le Clercq et al. 2014). It was reported that incomplete resection of polyps sized 5–20 mm ranged from 6.5 to 22.7% among endoscopists. Measurement of completeness of resection, however, is very difficult. To avoid incomplete resection, ESGE guidelines not only recommend using cold snare polypectomy for lesions sized 4 mm or larger but also recommend its use over cold biopsy forceps excision even for lesions sized 1–3 mm (Kaminski et al. 2017a; Ferlitsch et al. 2017).

7.3.7 Other Colonoscopy-Related Quality Issues

Some other quality issues pertaining to colonoscopy are worthwhile of mentioning. *Polyp retrieval rate* refers to the availability of polyp specimens for histological evaluation and it may impact whether further management is necessary (e.g., whether surgical intervention is necessary or determining recommendation on surveillance interval). The UK, Australian, and Irish programs all set the standard at 90% regarding polyp retrieval rate (S K. Guidelines for Quality Assurance in Colorectal Screening: National Screening Service 2017; Chilton 2011; Group.

TNBCSPQW 2009). *Comfort level* was also listed as a quality indicator of colonoscopy in some programs because it may affect the future screening compliance of the screenees. In UK program, reporting of comfort level using modified Gloucester comfort score descriptors is requested for all examinations (Chilton 2011). In Irish program, the standard was set at the level that 80% of the examinees with a comfort score of 1 or 2 from Gloucester Scale (Kelly et al. 2017). Surveillance colonoscopy may help to detect previously overlooked or newly developed neoplasm and provides additional protection against incident CRC thereby maximizing the effectiveness of screening. Appropriate and evidence-based surveillance intervals can balance between benefit (preventing incident CRC) and harm (complication and cost). In major guidelines, appropriate post-polypectomy surveillance recommendations are also listed as a quality indicator (Kaminski et al. 2017a). In the UK and Irish programs, attendance rate of surveillance colonoscopy is also a quality indicator and the standard is set at ≥85% of individuals scheduled for surveillance colonoscopy undergo the procedure within 3 months of scheduled date (Kelly et al. 2017; Chilton 2011).

7.4 Important Infrastructures for Quality Assurance

Some infrastructures are important and necessary for quality assurance in CRC screening program. First, central screening database accommodating important screening-related information, such as the number of screenees who are invited, number of FTI kit that delivered and returned, number of FIT with positive results, number of subjects who received colonoscopy after positive FIT, the number of subjects who had significant neoplasm at colonoscopy, the number of complication that occurred after colonoscopy, and so on. With such database, screening organizer is able to calculate the aforementioned important quality metrics thereby monitor and secure the performance of screening activity in each region. Second, in terms of colonoscopy quality, standardized colonoscopy reporting format is helpful for collecting important findings, output useful parameters, and finally link to effective interventions to improve quality. Many of the colonoscopy quality key performance indicators have been well established and validated at population level showing its impact on important clinical outcomes (incidence or mortality) and quality of life. For outputting these indicators, uniform, and well-designed endoscopy reporting system is required for systematic and uniform data registration via structured data entry of relevant information and endoscopic findings. By using this system, double data entry, which might result in mistakes, could be avoided and may be helpful for root cause analyses when post-colonoscopy complications or interval cancers occur afterward. In the Dutch program, a uniform colonoscopic reporting system was implemented from the beginning of the launch of their national screening program (van Doorn et al. 2014). It can not only enable endoscopists to create complete and standardized reports including all quality indicators but also facilitate regular production of standard analyses of all quality indicators for quality assurance and benchmarking at individual endoscopist, endoscopic unit, and screening program levels. In the Taiwanese program, a standardized and structured reporting format using dropdown menu was implemented in 2015. All units performing colonoscopy for FIT screening programs are obligated to use this standardized format and collected data is uploaded to central screening database. The screening organizer outputs the distribution of the colonoscopy quality metrics by plotting the performance of all units and demonstrating the placement of individual units (Fig. 7.2). Each unit receives this "transcript" annually as a feedback and uses it to facilitate identification of quality deficit thereby implementing specific training and education projects to improve colonoscopy quality. Finally, regional or national cancer registry system is indispensable for identifying and monitoring interval cancers (FIT interval cancers, PCCRC, or colonoscopy interval cancers). Because occurrence of interval cancer represents the deficit of the performance of screening, this may help to conduct root cause analyses at individual case level.

a

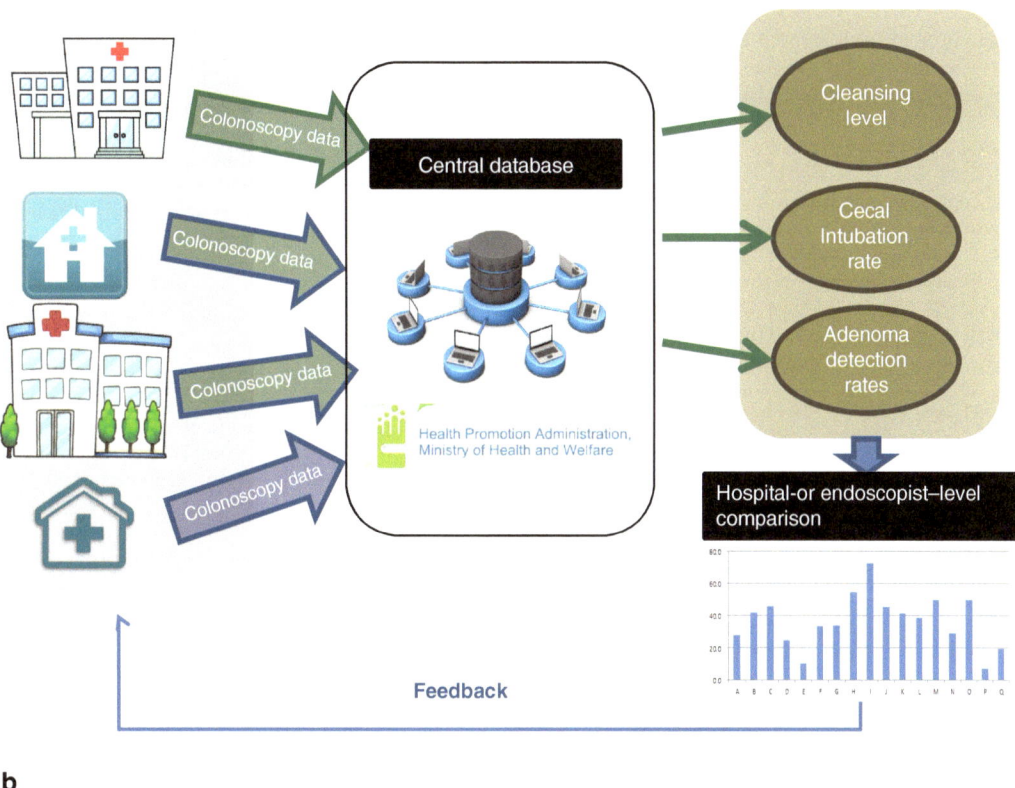

b

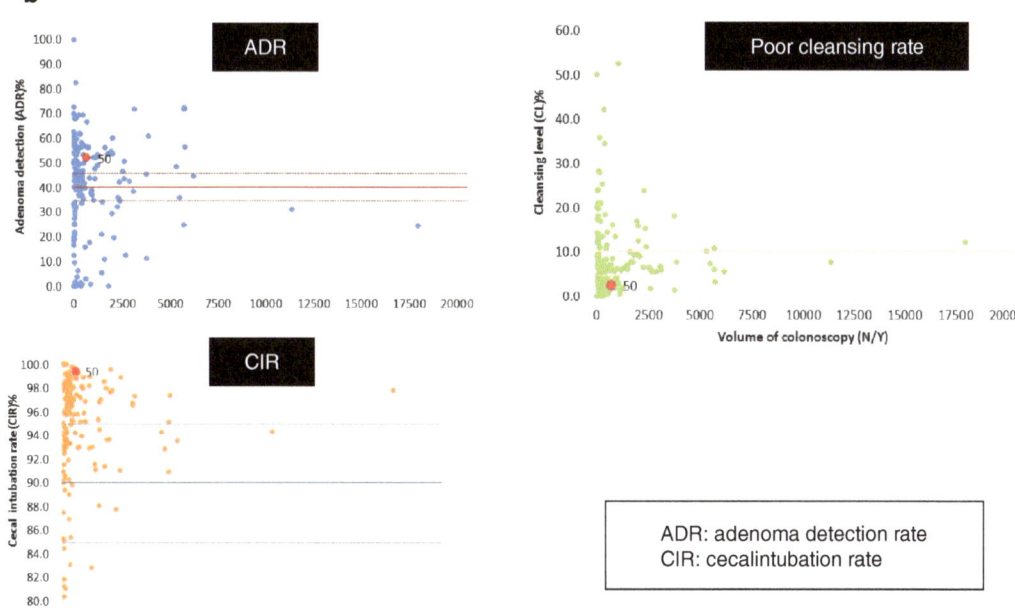

Fig. 7.2 (**a**) Framework of uploading colonoscopic findings by and feedback to individual endoscopic unit in Taiwan CRC Screening Program. (**b**) The "transcript" showing the distribution of colonoscopy quality metrics of all units and the placement of individual unit

References

Aniwan S, Orkoonsawat P, Viriyautsahakul V, et al. The secondary quality Indicator to improve prediction of adenoma miss rate apart from adenoma detection rate. Am J Gastroenterol. 2016;111:723–9.

ASGE Standards of Practice Committee; Saltzman JR, Cash BD, et al. Bowel preparation before colonoscopy. Gastrointest Endosc. 2015;81:781–94.

Australian Institute of Health and Welfare 2014. Key performance indicators for the National Bowel Cancer Screening Program: Technical report. Cancer series no. 87. Cat. no. CAN 84. Canberra: AIHW.

Baxter NN, Sutradhar R, Forbes SS, et al. Analysis of administrative data finds endoscopist quality measures associated with postcolonoscopy colorectal cancer. Gastroenterology. 2011;140:65–72.

Bernstein C, Thorn M, Monsees K, et al. A prospective study of factors that determine cecal intubation time at colonoscopy. Gastrointest Endosc. 2005;61:72–5.

BowelScreen. Guidelines for quality assurance in colorectal screening. Dublin: National Screening Service; 2017.

Brenner H, Tao S. Superior diagnostic performance of faecal immunochemical tests for haemoglobin in a head-to-head comparison with guaiac based faecal occult blood test among 2235 participants of screening colonoscopy. Eur J Cancer. 2013;49:3049–54.

Bronzwaer MES, Depla A, van Lelyveld N, et al. Quality assurance of colonoscopy within the Dutch national colorectal cancer screening program. Gastrointest Endosc. 2019;89:1–13.

Bucci C, Rotondano G, Hassan C, et al. Optimal bowel cleansing for colonoscopy: split the dose! A series of meta-analyses of controlled studies. Gastrointest Endosc. 2014;80:566–76. e2

Cha JM, Suh M, Kwak MS, et al. Risk of interval Cancer in fecal immunochemical test screening significantly higher during the summer months: results from the National Cancer Screening Program in Korea. Am J Gastroenterol. 2018;113:611–21.

Cheng SY, Li MC, Chia SL, et al. Factors affecting compliance with confirmatory colonoscopy after a positive fecal immunochemical test in a national colorectal screening program. Cancer. 2018;124:907–15.

Chiang TH, Chuang SL, Chen SL, et al. Difference in performance of fecal immunochemical tests with the same hemoglobin cutoff concentration in a nationwide colorectal cancer screening program. Gastroenterology. 2014;147:1317–26.

Chilton A et al. Quality assurance guidelines for colonoscopy. NHS BCSP Publ., 2011.

Chiu HM, Lin JT, Wang HP, et al. The impact of colon preparation timing on colonoscopic detection of colorectal neoplasms--a prospective endoscopist-blinded randomized trial. Am J Gastroenterol. 2006;101:2719–25.

Chiu HM, Chen SL, Yen AM, et al. Effectiveness of fecal immunochemical testing in reducing colorectal cancer mortality from the one million Taiwanese screening program. Cancer. 2015;121:3221–9.

Chiu SY, Chuang SL, Chen SL, et al. Faecal haemoglobin concentration influences risk prediction of interval cancers resulting from inadequate colonoscopy quality: analysis of the Taiwanese Nationwide colorectal Cancer screening program. Gut. 2017;66:293–300.

Choi NK, Lee J, Chang Y, et al. Acute renal failure following oral sodium phosphate bowel preparation: a nationwide case-crossover study. Endoscopy. 2014;46:465–70.

Chokshi RV, Hovis CE, Hollander T, et al. Prevalence of missed adenomas in patients with inadequate bowel preparation on screening colonoscopy. Gastrointest Endosc. 2012;75:1197–203.

Clark BT, Rustagi T, Laine L. What level of bowel prep quality requires early repeat colonoscopy: systematic review and meta-analysis of the impact of preparation quality on adenoma detection rate. Am J Gastroenterol. 2014;109:1714–23.

Colonoscopy quality standards and quality metrics in Taiwan. https://www.dest.org.tw/colonoscopy/content.asp?category=8&id=14

Cooper GS, Xu F, Barnholtz Sloan JS, et al. Prevalence and predictors of interval colorectal cancers in medicare beneficiaries. Cancer. 2012;118:3044–52.

Corley DA, Jensen CD, Marks AR, et al. Adenoma detection rate and risk of colorectal cancer and death. N Engl J Med. 2014;370:1298–306.

Corley DA, Jensen CD, Quinn VP, et al. Association between time to colonoscopy after a positive fecal test result and risk of colorectal Cancer and Cancer stage at diagnosis. JAMA. 2017;317:1631–41.

Ferlitsch M, Moss A, Hassan C, et al. Colorectal polypectomy and endoscopic mucosal resection (EMR): European Society of Gastrointestinal Endoscopy (ESGE) clinical guideline. Endoscopy. 2017;49:270–97.

Gavin DR, Valori RM, Anderson JT, et al. The national colonoscopy audit: a nationwide assessment of the quality and safety of colonoscopy in the UK. Gut. 2013;62:242–9.

Gohel TD, Burke CA, Lankaala P, et al. Polypectomy rate: a surrogate for adenoma detection rate varies by colon segment, gender, and endoscopist. Clin Gastroenterol Hepatol. 2014;12:1137–42.

Graser A, Stieber P, Nagel D, et al. Comparison of CT colonography, colonoscopy, sigmoidoscopy and faecal occult blood tests for the detection of advanced adenoma in an average risk population. Gut. 2009;58:241–8.

Greenspan M, Rajan KB, Baig A, et al. Advanced adenoma detection rate is independent of nonadvanced adenoma detection rate. Am J Gastroenterol. 2013;108:1286–92.

Harewood GC, Sharma VK, de Garmo P. Impact of colonoscopy preparation quality on detection of suspected colonic neoplasia. Gastrointest Endosc. 2003;58:76–9.

Hassan C, Rex DK, Zullo A, et al. Loss of efficacy and cost-effectiveness when screening colonoscopy is performed by nongastroenterologists. Cancer. 2012a;118:4404–11.

Hassan C, Giorgi Rossi P, Camilloni L, et al. Meta-analysis: adherence to colorectal cancer screening and the detection rate for advanced neoplasia, according to the type of screening test. Aliment Pharmacol Ther. 2012b;36:929–40.

Hassan C, East J, Radaelli F, et al. Bowel preparation for colonoscopy: European Society of Gastrointestinal Endoscopy (ESGE) guideline – update 2019. Endoscopy. 2019;51:775–94.

Hilsden RJ, Dube C, Heitman SJ, et al. The association of colonoscopy quality indicators with the detection of screen-relevant lesions, adverse events, and post-colonoscopy cancers in an asymptomatic Canadian colorectal cancer screening population. Gastrointest Endosc. 2015;82:887–94.

Hilsden RJ, Bridges R, Dube C, et al. Defining benchmarks for adenoma detection rate and adenomas per colonoscopy in patients undergoing colonoscopy due to a positive fecal immunochemical test. Am J Gastroenterol. 2016;111:1743–9.

Jaruvongvanich V, Sempokuya T, Laoveeravat P, et al. Risk factors associated with longer cecal intubation time: a systematic review and meta-analysis. Int J Color Dis. 2018;33:359–65.

Johnson DA, Barkun AN, Cohen LB, et al. Optimizing adequacy of bowel cleansing for colonoscopy: recommendations from the US multi-society task force on colorectal cancer. Gastroenterology. 2014;147:903–24.

Jover R, Herraiz M, Alarcon O, et al. Clinical practice guidelines: quality of colonoscopy in colorectal cancer screening. Endoscopy. 2012;44:444–51.

Kaminski MF, Regula J, Kraszewska E, et al. Quality indicators for colonoscopy and the risk of interval cancer. N Engl J Med. 2010;362:1795–803.

Kaminski MF, Thomas-Gibson S, Bugajski M, et al. Performance measures for lower gastrointestinal endoscopy: a European Society of Gastrointestinal Endoscopy (ESGE) quality improvement initiative. Endoscopy. 2017a;49:378–97.

Kaminski MF, Wieszczy P, Rupinski M, et al. Increased rate of adenoma detection associates with reduced risk of colorectal Cancer and death. Gastroenterology. 2017b;153:98–105.

Kelly S et al. Guidelines for Quality Assurance in Colorectal Screening, Second Edition. National Screening Service, Ireland., 2017.

le Clercq CM, Bouwens MW, Rondagh EJ, et al. Postcolonoscopy colorectal cancers are preventable: a population-based study. Gut. 2014;63:957–63.

Lebwohl B, Kastrinos F, Glick M, et al. The impact of suboptimal bowel preparation on adenoma miss rates and the factors associated with early repeat colonoscopy. Gastrointest Endosc. 2011;73:1207–14.

Lee JK, Liles EG, Bent S, et al. Accuracy of fecal immunochemical tests for colorectal cancer: systematic review and meta-analysis. Ann Intern Med. 2014;160:171.

Lee YC, Li Sheng Chen S, Ming-Fang Yen A, et al. Association between colorectal Cancer mortality and gradient fecal hemoglobin concentration in colonoscopy noncompliers. J Natl Cancer Inst. 2017;109:djw269.

Lee YC, Fann JC, Chiang TH, et al. Time to colonoscopy and risk of colorectal Cancer in patients with positive results from fecal immunochemical tests. Clin Gastroenterol Hepatol. 2019;17:1332–40. e3

Lo SH, Halloran S, Snowball J, et al. Colorectal cancer screening uptake over three biennial invitation rounds in the English bowel cancer screening programme. Gut. 2015;64:282–91.

Manes G, Amato A, Arena M, et al. Efficacy and acceptability of sodium picosulphate/magnesium citrate vs low-volume polyethylene glycol plus ascorbic acid for colon cleansing: a randomized controlled trial. Color Dis. 2013;15:1145–53.

Markowitz GS, Stokes MB, Radhakrishnan J, et al. Acute phosphate nephropathy following oral sodium phosphate bowel purgative: an underrecognized cause of chronic renal failure. J Am Soc Nephrol. 2005;16:3389–96.

Martel M, Barkun AN, Menard C, et al. Split-dose preparations are superior to day-before bowel cleansing regimens: a meta-analysis. Gastroenterology. 2015;149:79–88.

Meester RG, Doubeni CA, Lansdorp-Vogelaar I, et al. Variation in adenoma detection rate and the lifetime benefits and cost of colorectal Cancer screening: a microsimulation model. JAMA. 2015;313:2349–58.

Ministry of Helath. Labour, and Welfare of Japanese government. 第1回がん検診受診率等に関するワーキンググループ. プロセス指標、特に精検受診率基準値 の見直しについて. https://www.mhlw.go.jp/file/05-Shingikai-10901000-Kenkoukyoku-Soumuka/0000127231.pdf. 2016.

National Institute for Public Health and the Environment (RIVM) Monitoring and Evaluation of the Colorectal Cancer Screening 2018. https://www.rivm.nl/documenten/monitoring-and-evaluation-of-colorectal-cancer-screening-programme-2018

Park DI, Ryu S, Kim YH, et al. Comparison of guaiac-based and quantitative immunochemical fecal occult blood testing in a population at average risk undergoing colorectal cancer screening. Am J Gastroenterol. 2010;105:2017–25.

Park MJ, Choi KS, Lee YK, et al. A comparison of qualitative and quantitative fecal immunochemical tests in the Korean national colorectal cancer screening program. Scand J Gastroenterol. 2012;47:461–6.

Park SK, Kim HY, Lee CK, et al. Comparison of adenoma detection rate and adenoma per colonoscopy as a quality indicator of colonoscopy. Scand J Gastroenterol. 2016;51:886–90.

Parmar R, Martel M, Rostom A, et al. Validated scales for Colon cleansing: a systematic review. Am J Gastroenterol. 2016;111:197–204. quiz 205

Parra-Blanco A, Kaminaga N, Kojima T, et al. Colonoscopic polypectomy with cutting current: is it safe? Gastrointest Endosc. 2000;51:676–81.

Rabeneck L, Paszat LF, Saskin R, et al. Association between colonoscopy rates and colorectal cancer mortality. Am J Gastroenterol. 2010;105:1627–32.

Radaelli F, Paggi S, Hassan C, et al. Split-dose preparation for colonoscopy increases adenoma detection rate: a randomised controlled trial in an organised screening programme. Gut. 2017;66:270–7.

Rees CJ, Thomas Gibson S, Rutter MD, et al. UK key performance indicators and quality assurance standards for colonoscopy. Gut. 2016;65:1923–9.

Regev A, Fraser G, Delpre G, et al. Comparison of two bowel preparations for colonoscopy: sodium picosulphate with magnesium citrate versus sulphate-free polyethylene glycol lavage solution. Am J Gastroenterol. 1998;93:1478–82.

Reumkens A, Rondagh EJ, Bakker CM, et al. Post-colonoscopy complications: a systematic review, time trends, and meta-analysis of population-based studies. Am J Gastroenterol. 2016;111:1092–101.

Rex DK, Schoenfeld PS, Cohen J, et al. Quality indicators for colonoscopy. Gastrointest Endosc. 2015;81:31–53.

Rim JH, Youk T, Kang JG, et al. Fecal occult blood test results of the National Colorectal Cancer Screening Program in South Korea (2006–2013). Sci Rep. 2017;7:2804.

Robertson DJ, Lieberman DA, Winawer SJ, et al. Colorectal cancers soon after colonoscopy: a pooled multicohort analysis. Gut. 2014;63:949–56.

Robertson DJ, Lee JK, Boland CR, et al. Recommendations on fecal immunochemical testing to screen for colorectal neoplasia: a consensus statement by the US multi-society task force on colorectal Cancer. Gastroenterology. 2017;152:1217–37. e3

Rosen L, Bub DS, Reed JF 3rd, et al. Hemorrhage following colonoscopic polypectomy. Dis Colon Rectum. 1993;36:1126–31.

Ross WA, Thirumurthi S, Lynch PM, et al. Detection rates of premalignant polyps during screening colonoscopy: time to revise quality standards? Gastrointest Endosc. 2015;81:567–74.

Rutter MD, Beintaris I, Valori R, et al. World endoscopy organization consensus statements on post-colonoscopy and post-imaging colorectal Cancer. Gastroenterology. 2018;155:909–25. e3

Sanduleanu S, le Clercq CM, Dekker E, et al. Definition and taxonomy of interval colorectal cancers: a proposal for standardising nomenclature. Gut. 2015;64:1257–67.

Singh H, Nugent Z, Demers AA, et al. Rate and predictors of early/missed colorectal cancers after colonoscopy in Manitoba: a population-based study. Am J Gastroenterol. 2010a;105:2588–96.

Singh H, Nugent Z, Mahmud SM, et al. Predictors of colorectal cancer after negative colonoscopy: a population-based study. Am J Gastroenterol. 2010b;105:663–73. quiz 674

The National Bowel Cancer Screening Program Quality Working Group. Improving colonoscopy services in Australia. Australian Government Department of Health and Ageing, Canberra 2009.

van Doorn SC, van Vliet J, Fockens P, et al. A novel colonoscopy reporting system enabling quality assurance. Endoscopy. 2014;46:181–7.

Wang HS, Pisegna J, Modi R, et al. Adenoma detection rate is necessary but insufficient for distinguishing high versus low endoscopist performance. Gastrointest Endosc. 2013;77:71–8.

Wong JCT, Chiu HM, Kim HS, et al. Adenoma detection rates in colonoscopies for positive fecal immunochemical tests versus direct screening colonoscopies. Gastrointest Endosc. 2019;89:607–13. e1

Basic Theory of Screening for Short-Term Evaluation of Population-Based Screening for Colorectal Cancer

Hsiao-Hsuan Jen, Szu-Min Peng, Shu-Lin Chuang, and Chen-Yang Hsu

Abstract

Screening plays an important role in early detection of colorectal cancer (CRC) with an available screening tool followed by appropriate treatments and therapies to reach the ultimate goal of reducing colorectal cancer mortality given a progressive property of the evolution of CRC in the absence of screening. However, whether the effectiveness of screening in reducing mortality is highly dependent on when the uptake of screening is intervened at early or late time point of the duration between preclinical detectable phase (PCDP) and clinical phase (CP) estimated by the mean sojourn time (MST) dwelling at PCDP. The MST is cardinal estimate for the short-term evaluation of the quality control over the occurrence of interval cancers (cancers diagnosed between screens), a proxy for long-term effectiveness of population-based organized service screening.

In this chapter, we first introduce the basic screening theory from three-state evolution of CRC in terms of MST in relation to the time of screening. We proposed two methods to estimate the MST. The first prevalence pool method is illustrated with the UK randomized controlled trial on guaiac fecal occult blood test (gFOBT)-based screening program. The second day method, interval cancers as a percentage of the expected incidence with adjustment for MST, is revisited and modified to evaluate population-based organized service screening program in terms of test sensitivity, positive predictive value, and negative predictive value. Such a Day method is illustrated with the Taiwanese Colorectal Cancer Screening Programs with the screening tool of faecal immunochemical test (FIT). The proposed methodology on MST with a sound theory of screening is feasible for a short-term evaluation of population-based organized service screening to monitor the quality of service screening program and also reveal the odds of achieving long-term benefit of population-based screening for CRC.

H.-H. Jen · S.-M. Peng
Graduate Institute of Epidemiology and Preventive Medicine, College of Public Health, National Taiwan University, Taipei, Taiwan

S.-L. Chuang
Department of Medical Research, National Taiwan University Hospital, Taipei, Taiwan

C.-Y. Hsu (✉)
Graduate Institute of Epidemiology and Preventive Medicine, College of Public Health, National Taiwan University, Taipei, Taiwan

Master of Public Health Degree Program, National Taiwan University, Taipei, Taiwan

Keywords

Mean sojourn time · Sensitivity · Positive predictive value · Negative predictive value · Colorectal cancer screening

© Springer Nature Singapore Pte Ltd. 2021
H.-M. Chiu, H.-H. Chen (eds.), *Colorectal Cancer Screening*,
https://doi.org/10.1007/978-981-15-7482-5_8

Although it is of paramount importance to assess the effectiveness of population-based organized service screening for colorectal cancer (CRC), scientific evaluation is often hampered by four reasons. Firstly, there is a lacking of the comparator due to the property of service program offered for the entire target population. Second, the progressive nature of neoplastic disease also complicates the assessment of the efficacy of screening as demonstrated in Chap. 1 by using the epidemiological indicators of mortality and incidence of CRC because the uptake of screening may interrupt the disease natural history with early treatment and therapy. Third, the performance of the screening tool (sensitivity and specificity) can have impact on the effectiveness of screening program associated with the capability on identifying diseased subjects by the screening activity. Fourth, the primary endpoint for evaluation of the effectiveness mainly relies on CRC-specific mortality that often implicates the difficulty of logistics related to cost and time during a long-term follow-up.

In this chapter, we focus on the evaluation of population-based screening programs with short-term indicators making use of interval cancer. To provide a theoretically sound framework for the short-term evaluation of population-based organized service screening program, we first introduce the role of sojourn time in relation to the administration of screening and the time horizon of colorectal cancer progression in Sect. 8.1. The estimation and interpretation of mean sojourn time in the context of colorectal cancer screening are provided in Sect. 8.2. In Sect. 8.3, we introduce the concept of tool sensitivity and program sensitivity in the screening program taking into account the time dimension of colorectal cancer progression. The impact of sensitivity and specificity on the efficacy of screening program centering on interval cancer is illustrated in Sect. 8.4. We conclude with the application of such a basic screening theory for the short-term evaluation of fecal immunochemical test (FIT)-based Taiwan CRC Screening Program.

8.1 Disease Progression and Mean Sojourn Time Observed in Cancer Screening

Supported by a body of evidence on clinical and basic research, the evolution of CRC can be depicted by using a three-state progressive model, including the disease-free status, the micro disease state without symptoms (also called preclinical detectable phase abbreviated as PCDP), and the macro disease state with clinical symptoms of CRC (also called clinical phase abbreviated as CP). Based on the progressive property, detecting the asymptomatic micro disease state is the main target of organized service screening program. Embedded within the timeframe proposed by Walter and Day (1983), this three-state progressive model can be articulated with the intervention of screening for the detection of neoplastic lesion in the context of CRC evolution as shown in Fig. 8.1 that forms the backbone for the estimation on the duration of micro disease state (PCDP), a cardinal indicator for a short-term evaluation.

The time frame illustrated in Fig. 8.1 stems from the progressive process for CRC as elaborated as follows. An individual who is initially in a normal state (free of CRC) may progress into micro disease state without clinical symptoms (micro disease state) at time T1, corresponding to the time point of biological onset for tumor growth, i.e., initiation of the first abnormal clone. The state at T1 is usually undetectable with traditional screening methods, e.g., FIT used in colorectal cancer screening. As time goes by, the tumor will progress to T2, from which the cancer begins to become detectable by an available screening tool. If screening is not administered during this period, the disease will further develop to the macro disease state with clinical symptom at T3 which may results in a poorer prognosis compared with early and asymptomatic diseases detected by screening during its micro disease state. Screening is intended to find out those at insidi-

Fig. 8.1 Three-state disease progression model

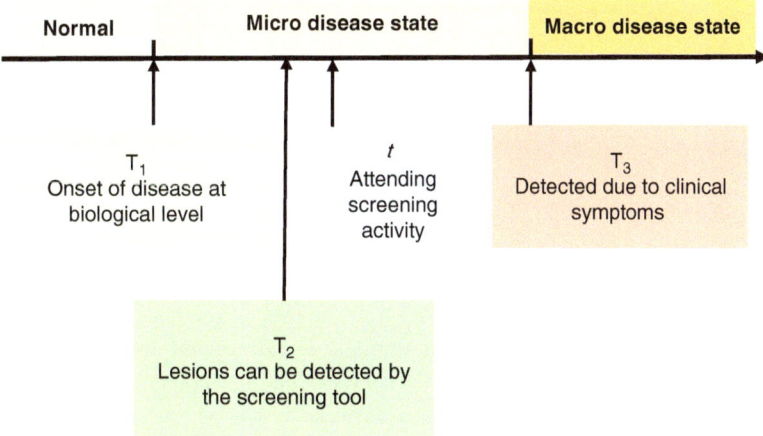

ous state of cancer (between T1 and T3, PCDP) before the progression to CP after T3. The time between T2 and T3 is the duration of PCDP, representing the period during which a subject remains in the microstate and can be detected by the available screening tool (PCDP).

8.2 Mean Sojourn Time in Screening Program

The time staying at the PCDP is often called the sojourn time. The average time dwelling in the asymptomatic state not only reflects the performance of screening tool in terms of early detection but also is crucial for the determination of inter-screening interval. Two methods of estimating the mean sojourn time for CRC screening program are introduced as follows.

8.2.1 The Concept of Prevalence Pool under the Context of Screen Theory

The concept of prevalence pool is depicted in Fig. 8.2 explained in detail as follows. Suppose a population with size N consists of m CRC cases detected in prevalent screen, which is equivalent to a cross-sectional survey with the prevalence (P) estimated by

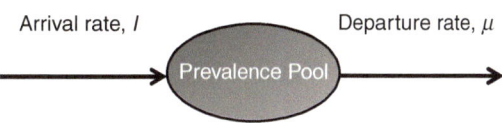

Fig. 8.2 The concept of prevalence pool considering the arrival rate (incidence rate of preclinical CRC) and departure rate (progression rate of preclinical CRC)

$$P = \frac{m}{N}. \tag{8.1}$$

In a steady population (i.e., inflow = outflow), we have the following balance equation in a small time inter (Δt)

$$I \times (N - m) \times \Delta t = \mu \times m \times \Delta t$$

$$\frac{m}{N - m} = \frac{I}{\mu} \tag{8.2}$$

Note that the arrival rate (I) as shown in Fig. 8.2 is equivalent to the incidence rate for asymptomatic CRC, which can only be detected through screening. Those with (the status of asymptomatic CRC will eventually progress to symptomatic phase and have departure from the prevalence pool of asymptomatic CRC. The departure rate μ is thus equivalent to the progression rate under the context of CRC evolution embedded within the screening program.

If $N \gg m$, $N - m \cong N$, the formula in (8.2) is thus simplified as follows:

$$P(\text{Prevalence}) = \frac{I(\text{Incidence})}{\mu}. \tag{8.3}$$

The average duration of dwelling in the status of asymptomatic CRC is thus derived by

$$\frac{P}{I} = \frac{1}{\mu} = \bar{D}\left(\text{Average Duration}\right) \quad (8.4)$$

This quantity is a proxy for estimating the mean sojourn time for CRC given the characteristics of population and also the tools used to detect asymptomatic lesions in the screening program. The mean sojourn time is used to denote the average duration of staying in asymptomatic PCDP status of CRC. We can estimate the survival function, $S(t)$, depicting the probability of dwelling in the asymptomatic status as a function of time by applying an exponential distribution with the parameter of μ.

$$S(t) = e^{-\mu t} \quad (8.5)$$

8.2.2 Applying the Prevalence Pool Method to the UK Trial on FOBT Screening

Between February, 1981, and January, 1991, 152,850 people aged 45–74 years who lived in the Nottingham area of the United Kingdom were recruited. Participants were randomly allocated FOB screening (7466) or no screening (controls; 76,384) (Hardcastle et al. 1996). With the available data on participants following up until June, 1995 (median follow-up of 7.8 years), a 15%

reduction in cumulative CRC mortality in the screening group (odds ratio 0.85 (95% CI 0.74–0.98) was observed.

The UK trial randomly allocated participants into either FOBT screening group ($n = 76,466$) or the control group ($n = 76,384$). In the screening group, 44,838 participants completed at least one screening. As an illustration, the estimation on the prevalence rate of preclinical CRC (P) and the background incidence rate (I) can be derived from the Tabular data. Note that all cancers appeared in a median follow-up of 7.8 years, which yielded the number of person-years in the screening and control groups, 597,944 and 596,396, respectively (Hardcastle et al. 1996).

The cancer rate at first screen, 2.1 per 1000, was higher than the expected underlying incidence rate (the control group), 1.44 (=856/596,369) per 1000 person-years. The incidence in subsequent screens (rounds 2–5 on average), 1.4 per 1000, was lower than the expected underlying incidence rate.

From the basic information listed above, the prevalence rate can be derived by

$$\text{Prevalence} = \frac{104}{44838} = 0.00232.$$

For the expected incidence rate of CRC, there are two approaches to obtain the estimate:

1. The expected underlying incidence rate from control group

$$\text{Expected incidence rate}\left(\text{control group}\right) = \frac{856}{596369} = 0.00144$$

Therefore, the P/I ratio can be estimated as

$$P \, / \, I \, \text{ratio} = \frac{0.00232}{0.00144} = 1.61 \, \text{yrs}$$

2. Subsequent screen + Interval cancer

$$\text{Expected incidence rate} = \frac{381}{348925\left(= \left[44838 - 104\right] \times 7.8\right)} = 0.00109$$

The P/I ratio in this approach is

$$P \, / \, I \, \text{ratio} = \frac{0.00232}{0.00109} = 2.13$$

This indicator, P/I ratio, means the average dwelling time of CRC from the preclinical detectable phase (PCDP) to the clinical phase (CP) is about 1.62–2.13 years.

8.3 Test Sensitivity, Program Sensitivity, and Disease Natural History

As a quality indicator, sensitivity is crucial for a screening program since a low sensitivity represents the scenario that a significant proportion of subjects with disease would be missed during screen and surface to the clinical phase later on (interval cancer). For a screening program with poor sensitivity or high proportion of interval cancer, the efficacy of mortality reduction would be compromised.

The traditional method to estimate sensitivity is based on the interval case approach, i.e., the ratio of screen-detected to screen-detected plus interval cancers. Although this method seems straightforward, the logic for this formula is unsound because the time aspect of early detection is ignored. The following shows why such a method is inappropriate for estimating the sensitivity in screening. Suppose a screen is carried out at t_1 as shown in Fig. 8.3. The sensitivity is usually defined as follows:

$$a / (a + c) \qquad (8.6)$$

based on the notation in Table 8.1.

Following the conventional definition on evaluating test accuracy, the specificity, positive predictive value (PPV), and negative predictive value (NPV) can be derived by

$$\mathrm{Sen} = P(T+ \mid D+) = \frac{a}{a+c}$$

$$\mathrm{Spe} = P(T- \mid D-) = \frac{d}{b+d}$$

$$\mathrm{PPV} = P(D+ \mid T+) = \frac{a}{a+b}$$

$$\mathrm{NPV} = P(D- \mid T+) = \frac{d}{c+d} \qquad (8.7)$$

However, both the frequency c and d are not available in the scenario of population-based screen since those with negative screening results will not go further to have confirmatory diagnosis and thus the true disease status is not exactly known.

To cope with this problem, an estimate, c^*, is obtained as the number of cases arising clinically in a short time interval after the screen. The time limit is usually set arbitrarily at 1 year after screening for cancer. The estimate of sensitivity is then:

$$\mathrm{Sensitivity} = \frac{a}{a + c^*}, \qquad (8.8)$$

where a is the number of screening-detected cancers and c^* is the number of false-negative cases (Day 1985).

The sensitivity can thus be derived using the ratio of incidence of interval cancer case to the expected incidence (I/E ratio) written as follows:

$$\mathrm{Sen} = 1 - \frac{I}{E}, \qquad (8.9)$$

where I is the incidence of interval cancer of the population attending screening program and E is the expected incidence of the population. Ideally,

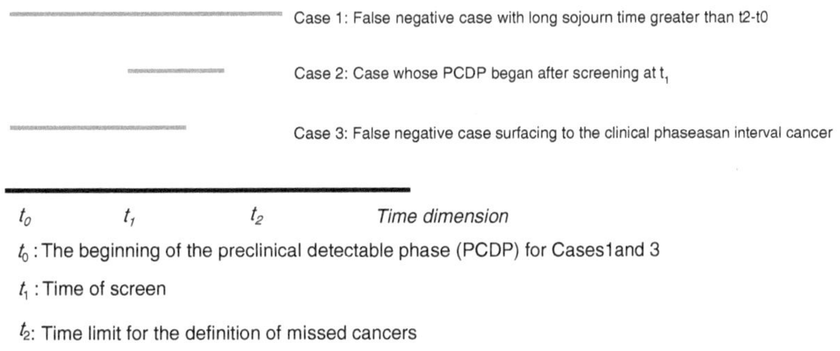

Fig. 8.3 Disease progression in relation to false-negative rate estimation using interval cancers in a set time period

Case 1: False negative case with long sojourn time greater than t2-t0

Case 2: Case whose PCDP began after screening at t$_1$

Case 3: False negative case surfacing to the clinical phaseasan interval cancer

t_0 t_1 t_2 Time dimension

t_0 : The beginning of the preclinical detectable phase (PCDP) for Cases1and 3

t_1 : Time of screen

t_2: Time limit for the definition of missed cancers

Table 8.1 Derivation of measurement error using the frequencies of test results (screening) by true disease status*

	True disease state (PCDP) Cancer	Cancer-free	Total
Screening(+)	a	b	$a + b = n_1$
Screening(−)	c	d	$c + d = n_0$
Total	$a + c$	$b + d$	$a + b + c + d = N$

*c and d are unavailable in population-based screening

the expected incidence can be derived from the passive screening population (control arm) for a randomized controlled trial. For the service screening program, the choice of E should represent the underlying incidence of the population attending screening program.

8.4 Sensitivity and Specificity in Screening Program

8.4.1 Estimate the Sensitivity in the Screening Program

Although the expression in (8.8) contains an estimate of false-negative cases, the logic is wrong because c^* also included those cancers with very short preclinical detectable phase (PCDP), which entered the PCDP after the screen. Consequently, using the formula of (8.9) to estimate sensitivity is subject to the assumption that all of interval cases are from false-negative cases. However, three types of cancers should be considered while taking into account the time dimension from the PCDP to the clinical phase (CP). As shown in Fig. 8.3, colorectal cancers arising after a negative screen will be made up of both false-negative cases ("Case 1" and "Case 3" of Fig. 8.3) and those cases whose PCDP began after the screening test ("Case 2" of Fig. 8.3), with the duration of PCDP less than t_2-t_1. The estimate of sensitivity based on expression (8.8) ignores the false-negative cases with sojourn time greater than t_2-t_0 ("Case 1" of Fig. 8.3) and includes those such as "Case 2" of Fig. 8.3. The biological characteris-

tics of these three types of cases are summarized as follows:

Case 1: Truly false-negative case at t_1, but *not been observed* as interval cancer. This case was missed at the screening t_1 but remained symptomatic until t_2. The time staying at the PCDP was greater than t_2-t_0.

Case 2: Newly developed rapid progressive cancer observed as an *interval cancer*. This case has the PCDP commencing after screen(t_1) and surfacing to the CP before t_2. The time from PCDP to CP was shorter than t_2-t_1.

Case 3: Truly false-negative case at t_1, and observed as an interval cancer. This case was in the PCDP at screening at t_1 but missed. The PCDP was longer than t_1-t_0 but shorter than t_2-t_0.

The traditional proportional incidence method takes Case 2 and Case 3 into account in the calculation of c^*. By including Case 2, the fast progression with a short PCDP, it may lead to overestimation of c^*. By excluding Case 1, the slow progression with a long PCDP, this method may underestimate c^*. Therefore, this method is potentially associated with the risks of underestimation or overestimation of the test sensitivity. The biased estimation is related to the distribution of sojourn time (PCDP).

A refinement to this is to take c^* with only those tumors arising during this time period t_2-t_1, which an expert panel or independent radiologist has classified as missed on reviewing the screening mammograms. In principle, this eliminates those tumors entering the PCDP after screening, but it does not capture those tumors which were missed at the time of screening but surface to clinical phase after t_2. It also has a subjective element that may not be universally acceptable. For example, if the screening radiologist missed a tumor, the expert panel or independent radiologist may also do so. The argument indicated above suggests that the program sensitivity in relation to screening is strongly dependent on sojourn time and screening interval. The sensitivity would be high if the disease has a longer sojourn time and short screening interval. Thus, Day proposed a method to estimate the sensitivity which is based on the distribution of sojourn time and the expected incidence in the absence of screening.

8.4.2   Mathematical Formula for Interval Cancer

To approach this problem, it is necessary to adjust the variation of PCDP by taking into consideration the sojourn time of all three cases (NE Day 1985). When $F(t)$ is defined as the probability distribution function of the sojourn time, I as the incidence of CRC, and S as the sensitivity of the screening test, the observed numbers of interval cancer can be given by:

$$E \times (1-S) \times \int_0^T \left[1 - F(t) \right] dt \qquad (8.10)$$

for Case 1 and Case 3, and

$$E \times \int_0^T F(t) dt \qquad (8.11)$$

for Case 2.

During the following time T, the observed incidence rate of interval cancer (I) is the sum of the above cases divided by T and written as follows:

$$I = E \times (1-S) \times \frac{1}{T} \int_0^T \left[1 - F(t) \right] dt + E \times \frac{1}{T} \int_0^T F(t) dt$$

$$= E - E \times S + E \times S \times \frac{1}{T} \int_0^T F(t) dt. \quad (8.12)$$

Therefore, as proposed by Day in 1985, the test sensitivity adjusting for sojourn time distribution in the denominator can be given by

$$S = \frac{1 - I/E}{1 - \frac{1}{T} \int_0^T F(t) dt}. \qquad (8.13)$$

Assuming the probability distribution of the sojourn time as exponential, the above equation can be simplified as follows:

$$S = \frac{1 - I/E}{1 - \frac{1}{T} \int_0^T \left[1 - e^{-\lambda t} \right] dt} = \frac{\lambda \times T \times (E - I)}{E \times \left(1 - e^{-\lambda t} \right)}. (8.14)$$

Following the time dynamic concept depicted as above, specificity in screen program can be estimated as

$$\frac{d^*}{b + d^*} \qquad (8.15)$$

where $d^* = n_0 - c^*$.

8.4.3   Positive and Negative Predictive Values

Positive predictive value is the proportion of subjects with a positive result after screening among those who have the underlying disease. In the theory of screening, it is an indicator for estimating the proportion of screen-detected tumors that would have surfaced to clinical cases had no screening been offered. Predictive value is determined by three estimates, test specificity, prevalence of PCDP, and test sensitivity. A low positive predictive value gives a clue to low specificity or low prevalence of disease. When time dimension is incorporated an estimate of predictive value would be affected by both sojourn time and test sensitivity. Over-detected cases may be indexed by a long sojourn time. The estimate of sensitivity would be affected when the interval case approach is adopted.

PPV is a specific measure for the yield of cancer screening. Note that it is not the same as the predictive value that is used for biopsy for confirming malignancy. It estimates the proportion of tumors detected at the prevalent screen that would have been diagnosed as symptomatic clinical cases had screening been not offered. Under this context, the predictive value is therefore defined as the proportion of true positives at first screen wherein overdiagnosed cases are more likely to occur. It is therefore consistent with the definition of PPV in terms of diagnostic methods (Duffy et al. 1996).

A two-stage procedure is often used to (1) estimate the mean sojourn time (MST) assuming 100% sensitivity and specificity, and then to (2) calculate the sensitivity and PPV.

$$PPV = \frac{EP\left(= E \times S \times MST\right)}{P} \quad (8.16)$$

PPV   Positive predictive value.
E   The Expected incidence in the absence of
       screening.
S   Sensitivity.
EP   The expected prevalence of cancers.
P   Prevalence at the first screen.

In a similar vein, the negative predictive value (NPV) in screen program can be estimated by

$$NPV = \frac{1-EP}{1-P} \quad (8.17)$$

Table 8.2 Sensitivity (%) and false-positive rate at different cutoffs of FIT value

Cutoff	Sensitivity (95% CI)	False-positive rate (95% CI)
30	84.6 (73.7–91.5)	22.9 (22.4–23.4)
50	81.5 (70.2–89.2)	12.9 (12.5–13.4)
70	81.5 (70.2–89.2)	8.5 (8.2–8.9)
90	81.5 (70.2–89.2)	6.4 (6.1–6.8)
100	81.5 (70.2–89.2)	5.7 (5.4–6.0)
110	80.0 (68.5–88.0)	5.2 (4.9–5.5)
130	72.3 (60.3–81.8)	4.3 (4.1–4.6)
150	69.2 (57.1–79.2)	3.8 (3.5–4.0)
170	64.6 (52.3–75.2)	3.3 (3.1–3.5)
190	64.6 (52.3–75.2)	3.0 (2.8–3.2)

8.5 Application of Basic Screening Theory to Fecal Immunochemical Test-based Colorectal Cancer Screening in Taiwan

8.5.1 Sensitivity of Fecal Immunochemical Test with Varying Cutoff

Although positive result of FIT was defined as 100 ng Hb/mL buffer (equivalent to 20 μg Hb/g feces) in Keelung Community-based Integrated Screening Program (KCIS), a quantitative value of FIT was demonstrated in a dose-response manner when biological gradient between f-Hb concentration and incidence of colorectal neoplasm was corroborated in the previous study (Chen et al. 2007). The study design for such a quantitative assessment between the value of FIT and the ascertainment of CRC is presented in Fig. 8.1 of the original literature of Chen et al. in 2007. The biological gradient of f-Hb concentration was classified at the prevalent screen. Those who had f-Hb ≥100 ng Hb/mL buffer were defined as positive and were then confirmed with colonoscopy for the referrals or ascertained through the linkage of positive subjects refusing to undergo confirmatory diagnosis with a nationwide cancer registry during the follow-up period. Regarding those with the value of FIT below 100, CRC cases were also ascertained in a similar manner making use of the nationwide cancer registry.

A series of results on sensitivity, false-positive and odds of being affected given a positive result (OAPR) are shown in Table 8.2. Table 8.2 also shows a string of cutoffs of f-Hb from 30 to 200 (ng Hb/mL buffer) using data derived from KCIS. The area under ROC (AUROC) curve was 87% (95% CI: 81–93%). The optimal cutoff was noted at 100 ng Hb/mL buffer with the corresponding figures of sensitivity, false-positive, and OAPR for detection of CRC equal to 81.5% (95% CI:70.2–89.2%), 5.7% (95% CI: 5.4–6.0%), and 1.24 (1.19–1.32) (Table 8.2). The threshold value was 110 ng Hb/mL buffer for women given 89% (95% CI: 80%–98%), Chen et al. 2007) of AUROC curve. The corresponding threshold value for men was 100 ng/m given 87% (95%CI: 80%–95%) of AUROC curve. The overlapping result of 95% CIs of AUROC curve indicates that the selection of cutoff would not vary with gender (Chen et al. 2007).

8.5.2 FIT Sensitivity for CRC Screening in KCIS, Taiwan

Although the incidence of colorectal cancer (CRC) has been increasing in the majority of intermediate-risk countries, whether to implement mass screening is still subject to the trade-off between costs and low yield. To this end, a multiple disease screening approach was envisaged to cover FIT. In the Keelung multiple disease screening programs, annual FIT were offered for 26,008 screenees between 2000 and 2002.

Table 8.3 Incidence rate of CRC after a negative screening result, as a percentage of the incidence in the absence of screening, Keelung program

Age at entry (years)	Interval cancers	Person-years	Interval cancer rate (I)[a]	Expected incidence (E)[a]	I/E (%)	Sensitivity (1-I/E, %)
Overall	11	28,282.71	38.89	130.93	30	70
50–59	1	10,807.27	9.25	48.14	19	81
60–69	3	10,642.00	28.19	138.44	20	80
70–79	7	6833.44	102.44	273.16	38	62

Modified from Kuo-Ching Yang et al., Colorectal cancer screening with faecal occult blood test within a multiple disease screening programme: an experience from Keelung, Taiwan. J Med Screen. 2006;13 Suppl 1:S8–13
[a]per 100,000 person-years

Table 8.4 Comparisons of the number of interval cancer, interval cancer rate, and test sensitivity between 2 quantitative fecal immunochemical tests

	Person-year at risk	No. of ICs	Incidence of IC (expected incidence in the absence of screening)[a]	Proportional incidence	1-proportional incidence, % (95% CI)	Test sensitivity, % (95% CI)
FIT 1						
50–59 years	936,177	182	19.4 (62.9)	0.31	69 (64–75)	81 (74–88)
60–69 years	564,452	278	49.3 (152.6)	0.32	68 (63–72)	80 (74–85)
Total	1,500,629	460	30.7 (96.6)	0.32	68 (65–72)	80 (76–84)
FIT 2						
50–59 years	196,885	55	27.9 (62.9)	0.44	56 (47–66)	65 (55–78)
60–69 years	118,536	73	61.6 (152.6)	0.40	60 (52–69)	71 (61–82)
Total	315,421	128	40.6 (96.6)	0.42	58 (52–65)	68 (61–76)

IC interval cancer
Modified from Tsung-Hsien Chiang, et al., Difference in Performance of Fecal Immunochemical Tests With the Same Hemoglobin Cutoff Concentration in a Nationwide Colorectal Cancer Screening Program. Gastroenterology 2014;147:1317–1326
[a]Per 100,000 person-years at risk

Using the proportionate incidence method, the overall sensitivity of KCIS program between 2000 and 2002 was 70% (1–30%, see Table 8.3). The corresponding figures for three age groups were 81% for 50–59 years, 80% for 60–69 years, and 62% for 70–79 years (Yang et al. 2006).

8.5.3 Sensitivity of National Colorectal Cancer Screening Program in Taiwan

In our nationwide screening program, 956,005 Taiwanese residents aged 50–69 years would be invited from 2004 through 2009. Of them, 78% (n = 747,076) were screened with FIT1, the OC-Sensor test (Eiken Chemical Co, Tokyo, Japan). The remaining 22% (n = 208,929) were screened with FIT2, the HM-Jack test (Kyowa Medex Co Ltd., Tokyo, Japan). A standardized reporting unit system gave 20 μg Hb/g feces of the cutoff for defining positive results. Chiang et al. evaluated the performance of the two screening tools based on the nationwide CRC screening program in Taiwan (Chiang et al. 2014).

Basic results on the frequency and the rate of interval cancer and test sensitivity two types of FIT tests (FIT1 and FIT2) are summarized in Table 8.4. Two approaches are also attempted here, including proportional incidence method and the test sensitivity making allowance for sojourn time. As far as FIT1 is concerned, the mean sojourn time, the inverse of the progression rate form PCDP to CP (equal to 0.327 per year) for CRC staying in the PCDP was 3 years or so. Given one-year of following up false-negative cases that surface clinical symptoms from the time since last negative screen, the interval cancer rate (I) was estimated as 30.7 per 10^5 person-years. Suppose the expected incidence rate in the absence of screening (E) was 96.6 per 10^5 person-years, the test sensitivity with adjustment for sojourn time was estimated as 80% (see Table 8.4). In a similar fashion, the corresponding test sensitivity for FIT2 was 68% based on 40.6 per 10^5 of interval cancer rate given the identical figures of the mean sojourn time and the expected incidence rate.

In theory, screening plays a vital role in early detection of colorectal cancer that in turn leads to the reduction of colorectal cancer mortality. However, whether the effectiveness of screening in reducing mortality is determined by when the uptake of screening is intervened at the time point of between pre-clinical detectable phase (PCDP) and clinical phase (CP). The theory of screening for estimating the distribution of the mean sojourn time (MST) dwelling at PCDP is therefore of paramount importance. The MST forms a cardinal estimate for the short-term evaluation of the quality control over the reduction of interval cancers (cancers diagnosed between screens), a proxy for long-term effectiveness of population-based organized service screening.

The basic screening theory based on the three-state evolution of CRC in terms of MST in relation to the time of screening is first introduced. We proposed two methods to estimate the MST. The first simple method with the concept of the prevalence pool is illustrated with the UK randomized controlled trail for guaiac faecal occult blood test (gFOBT)-based screening program to demonstrate its usefulness. The second Day method under the concept of interval cancers as a percentage of the expected incidence with adjustment for MST, is revisited and

modified to evaluate the test sensitivity of the screening tool applied to population-based organized service screening program and its derivatives of positive predictive value and negative predictive value. Such a Day method is illustrated with the FIT-based Taiwan Colorectal Cancer Screening Programs. The proposed methodology on MST with the sound theory of screening is very useful for providing evidence on the short-term effectiveness of population-based organized service screening. So doing offers three merits for evaluation of population-based organized service screening program while waiting for the results of CRC mortality and also providing The advantages of the proposed methodology may tackle the problem without the control group, dispense with long-term follow-up, and provide an insight into the evaluation of long-term effectiveness of population-based organized service screening program that will be delineated in Chap. 9.

References

Chen LS, Liao CS, Chang SH, Lai HC, Chen THH. Cost-effectiveness analysis for determining optimal cut-off of immunochemical fecal occult blood test for population-based colorectal Cancer screening (KCIS 16). J Med Screening. 2007;14(4):191–9.

Chiang TH, et al. Difference in performance of fecal immunochemical tests with the same hemoglobin cutoff concentration in a nationwide colorectal cancer screening program. Gastroenterology. 2014;147(6):1317–26.

Day NE. Estimating the sensitivity of a screening test. J Epidemiol Community Health. 1985 Dec;39(4):364–6.

Duffy SW, Chen THH, Tabar L, Fagerberg G, Paci E. Sojourn time, sensitivity, and positive predictive value of mammography screening of breast cancer in women aged under 50. Int JEpidemiol. 1996;25:1139–45.

Hardcastle JD, et al. Randomised controlled trial of faecal-occult-blood screening for colorectal cancer. Lancet. 1996;348(9040):1472–7.

Walter SD, Day NE. Estimation of the duration of a pre-clinical disease state using screening data. Am J Epidemiol. 1983;118(6):865–86.

Yang K-C, et al. Colorectal cancer screening with fecal occult blood test within a multiple disease screening program: an experience from keelung, Taiwan. J Med Screen. 2006;13(Suppl 1):8–13.

Evaluating Population-Based Colorectal Cancer Screening Beyond a Randomized Controlled Trial: A Mathematical Modelling Approach

9

Amy Ming-Fang Yen and Hsiu-Hsi Chen

Abstract

Although the effectiveness of mass screening for colorectal cancer (CRC), stool-based tests, for example, has been demonstrated by randomized controlled trials (RCTs), whether the same benefits can be similarly observed in population-based organized service screening programs is subject to multiple factors and a complex multistate disease process. Elucidating the natural history of multistate CRC with a mathematical modelling approach can provide an opportunity to test various scenarios involved in population-based organized service screening programs. We first provide rationales and unique characteristics of the modelling approach in contrast to the traditional analysis. We then reviewed a series of stochastic models applied to elucidate the natural history of the disease and to evaluate screening programs for colorectal cancer in the literature. These models cover the traditional homogeneous Markov model, the non-homogeneous Markov model, and the semi-Markov model. We also demonstrate how the temporal natural history of the disease modeled by the underlying stochastic processes can be applied to different scenarios, including a case-cohort sampling design for elucidating the disease course of adenoma carcinoma pathway, assessment of the efficacy of reducing malignant transformation and the effectiveness of population-based screening programs, decision analysis, and health economic decision models. A mathematical modelling approach is an efficient alternative method for evaluating a series of subsidiary issues of population-based organized service screening dispensing with a randomized controlled trial study or a complex quasi-experimental study that requires the comparator.

Keywords

Disease natural history · Effectiveness Evaluation · Markov model · Screening policy

A. M.-F. Yen (✉)
School of Oral Hygiene, College of Oral Medicine, Taipei Medical University, Taipei, Taiwan
e-mail: amyyen@tmu.edu.tw

H.-H. Chen
Institute of Epidemiology and Preventive Medicine, College of Public Health, National Taiwan University, Taipei, Taiwan

© Springer Nature Singapore Pte Ltd. 2021
H.-M. Chiu, H.-H. Chen (eds.), *Colorectal Cancer Screening*,
https://doi.org/10.1007/978-981-15-7482-5_9

9.1 Rationales for Evaluating a Population-Based Colorectal Cancer Screening Program beyond Randomized Controlled Trials

Population-based cancer organized service screening for colorectal cancer (CRC) has increasingly gained attention in recent years, particularly in Asian regions, on the grounds of four reasons. First, a series of randomized controlled trials (RCTs) in Western countries have already demonstrated the effectiveness of screening in reducing mortality and possibly incidence (Mandel et al. 1993; Hardcastle et al. 1996; Kronborg et al. 1996). Second, people in the public health domain are faced with the challenge of increasing time trends of the incidence rates of CRC over the past two decades. Third, health decision makers under the auspices of health authorities in each region are intended to detect early-stage cancers so as to improve the survival of CRCs. Fourth, with the advent of new medical technology and treatments and therapies pertinent to CRC, how can they be applied to clinical surveillance of early-detected cancers for improving the prognosis of death from CRC is worthy of being investigated.

Although the previous RCTs on CRC screening have shown statistically significant results on mortality reduction, these findings may not be generalized to other countries with similar but service-oriented screening programs. Moreover, these RCTs may tell whether the uptake of screening can work but it may not throw light on why and how they can work particularly when they are applied to a population-based organized service screening program. The effectiveness of a population-based screening program for CRC is highly determined by a constellation of factors that are classified into two parts. The first includes basic screening characteristics (such as screening attendance rate, colonoscopy referral rate, and colonoscopy quality), temporal disease natural history, and the performance of the screening tools. The second part pertains to the clinical surveillance of precursors of invasive carcinoma and treatment modalities of early-detected cancers. The former plays a crucial role in the determination of screening policies such as age to begin with screening and age to stop screening, inter-screening interval, and the choice of screening tool. The latter plays a crucial role in the prognosis of screen-detected CRCs. It should be noted that the way to evaluate the effectiveness of these service screening programs would be distinct from that to evaluate the RCT.

Evaluating an organized service screening program is vulnerable to the influence of confounding factors, selection bias, and misclassifications of being exposed to screening and the ascertainment of the outcome. Although a number of studies focusing on the evaluation of effectiveness in reducing mortality among those organized service screening programs have shown how to make adjustment for certain bias such as self-selection resulting from the volunteer participating in an organized service screening (Chiu et al. 2015), factors affecting the effectiveness of a population-based service screening program are manifold and the disease process also involves a multistep progression, it is of paramount importance to provide a systematic evaluation of the effectiveness of an organized service screening based on a further sophisticated statistical model such as a multistate stochastic model.

9.2 Design, Data, and Conventional Analysis for Evaluation

9.2.1 Quasi-experimental Study Design

As mentioned before, the effectiveness of mass screening using a randomized controlled design might not have the same benefits as that of population-based organized service screening programs with a quasi-experimental design because the related factors or parameters cannot be appropriately regulated or well controlled with a good quality-assurance program.

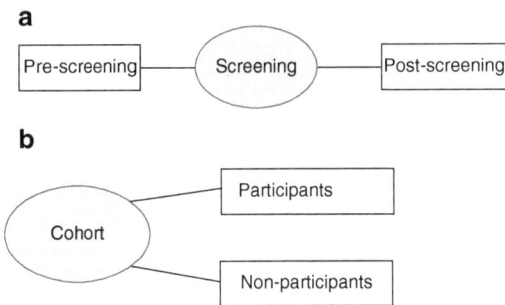

Fig. 9.1 Two quasi-experimental designs of population-based service screening program. (**a**) One-group pretest–posttest design. (**b**) Posttest-only nonequivalent design

Figure 9.1 illustrates two quasi-experimental designs, the one-group pretest–posttest design and the posttest-only nonequivalent design. The one-group pretest–posttest design for the evaluation of the cancer screening program compares the primary outcome such as mortality of the entire eligible population in the period prior to screening (pre-screen period) with that after screening (post-screen period). Cancer cases and the associated subsequent deaths were ascertained for each period to compare the survival or mortality from cancer between the two groups. The second design, which is named the posttest-only nonequivalent design, adopts a contemporaneous unscreened group composed of those who were invited to the screening but refused to attend (unexposed group).

9.2.1.1 Data Sources for Evaluation

To conduct the evaluation of population-based service screening for CRC, it is ideal to make use of registry data comprehensively representing the underlying incidence and mortality associated with CRC. Four specific registry systems and their application are delineated as follows:

1. Population registry.
   Population registry is used to calculate person-years of the invited and uninvited group to further calculate the screening coverage rate and attendance rate.
2. Mass screening registry.
   Individualized screening history consisting of prevalent screen and subsequent screens

and the numerator of individual screen-detected cases ascertained in each round of screen can be obtained from the mass screen registry.
3. Cancer registry.
   Individual data on interval cancers and cancers derived from non-attendees can be ascertained by linking the screened cohort with the cancer registry.
4. Death registry.
   Individual data on date and cause of death enables us to determine the mortality rates associated with CRC in the invited and uninvited groups.

9.2.1.2 Computer-aided System of Evaluation of a Screening Program

Chen et al. (2010) developed a graphic interface system, the Computer-aided System of Evaluation for Population-based All-in-One Service Screening (CASE-PASS), with SAS/AF software in a pull-down menu style, running on an SAS platform. This system underpins the two above-mentioned experimental designs, the posttest-only nonequivalent design, and the one-group pretest–posttest design. The system includes three major analyses: cumulative mortality analysis, survival analysis with lead-time adjustment, and self-selection bias adjustment.

Although data on year of diagnosis, year of death, age at diagnosis, death from a specific cancer, and exposure to the screen are required, aggregate data are sufficient for the denominator of person-years if individual data on the history of screen are not available.

9.3   A Modelling Approach to Evaluating Colorectal Cancer Screening

In addition to the conventional method for evaluation of population-based service screening program, there is an alternative to evaluate the effectiveness of population-based service screening program with a modeling approach. The main idea is to apply a mathematic model to quantify disease natural history in the absence of screening for forming the control group and then to assess how various screening policies and modalities can be administered to alter the disease's natural history.

Although the efficacy of screening for CRC has been demonstrated by population-based RCTs, as evidenced by a 15–33% mortality reduction when the biennial guaiac–fecal occult blood test (gFOBT) was adopted in Europe and the United States (Hardcastle et al. 1996; Kronborg et al. 1996; Mandel et al. 1993), such results cannot be directly applied to countries with low and intermediate incidence rates of CRC or to scenarios in which different screening modalities, such as primary sigmoidoscopy and colonoscopy, are proposed. It is also impractical to conduct another RCT for every new scenario. However, observational studies, such as case-control studies, have been often criticized for the potential biases. Identifying a fair comparison (control) group is the key to obtaining the unbiased estimate of the efficacy of screening.

The advantage of using such a modelling approach may also outweigh the benefits of the use of RCTs, particularly when the number of arms in a randomized controlled trial is too excessive for gaining sufficient statistical power. Modelling disease natural history can also provide an opportunity to test various screening policies, including different inter-screening interval, different age of commencing and terminating screening, and different kinds of detection modalities (embracing multiple detection modalities).

In this section, we reviewed a series of stochastic models applied to elucidate the disease's natural history and evaluate screening programs for CRC in the literature. These models cover the traditional homogeneous Markov model, the non-homogeneous Markov model, and the semi-Markov model.

Table 9.1 shows a series of stochastic models in the literature that have been developed for the evaluation of screening programs for CRC.

9.3.1 Multistate Process of CRC with the Homogeneous Markov Model

The three-state Markov model delineating the disease process into three stages (CRC-free, preclinical detectable phase (PCDP), and clinical phase (CP)) has been proposed to quantify the temporal disease natural history of cancer. Owing to the multistate property, the Markov model can estimate an occult transition, such as PCDP to CP, based on data from different detection modes, including disease-free at screening (CRC-free→CRC-free), screen-detected cancer (CRC-free→PCDP), and interval cancers (CRC-free→CP). In addition, the simultaneous estimation of both the incidence of preclinical cancer and the mean sojourn time (MST, the inverse of the transition rate from PCDP to CP under the Markovian property) could be used to study the dependence between the two different transition rates.

Chen et al. (1999) applied the Markov model to a selective screening program in a multicenter screening program for CRC for high-risk group subjects in the Taiwan Multicenter Cancer Screening (TAMCAS) project. In their analysis, the preclinical incidence rate was estimated as 4 (95% CI: 2.9–5.0) per 1000, accompanied by 2.85-year MST (95% CI: 2.15–4.30). They also incorporated sensitivity into their model and estimated the sensitivity of colonoscopy in combination with fecal occult blood test (FOBT) or double-contrast barium enema for this high-risk group as 94.98% (95% CI: 24.36–99.91%).

Elucidation of disease natural history of cancer by clinical stages in the PCDP and CP enables one to assess the possibility of a screening benefit. As Dukes' stage plays an important role in the prognosis of CRC, Wong et al. (2004) showed particular interest in the progression rate of CRC by Dukes' stage using a five-state Markov model (CRC-free, PCDP Dukes' AB, PCDP Dukes' CD, CP Dukes' AB, and CP Dukes' CD) applied to the TAMCAS. They found that the relative transition rate (RTR) from PCDP Dukes' AB to

Table 9.1 Literature on modeling disease natural history of colorectal cancer by using multistate Markov models

Author, year	Study	Markov models	CRC-free -> PCDP CRC	CRC-free -> Diminutive adenoma	Diminutive - > Small adenoma	Small - > Large adenoma	Large adenoma - > PCDP AB	Large adenoma - > CRC	PCDP - CP > CRC	PCDP AB- > PCDP CD	PCDP AB- > CP AB	PCDP AB- > CP CD	Sensitivity
Chen et al. (1999)	TAMCAS, high-risk group screening	3-state Markov model	0.004						0.3513				94.98%
Wong et al. (2004)	TAMCAS, high-risk group screening	5-state nonhomogeneous Markov model	Weibull $(1.45*10^{-5}, 2.2824)$							0.2955	0.2095	0.5216	78.74%
Yang et al. (2006)	Community-based program	8-state Markov model		0.0013	0.0696	0.1854	0.1772			0.3079	0.2455	0.9241	
Chen et al. (2003)	Case-cohort study	5-state Markov model		0.0031	0.038	0.13		0.19					
Chiu et al. (2011)	Meta-analysis from RCTs	5-state Markov model	0.00148							0.28	0.22	0.72	

*AB: Duke's stage A and B; CD: Duke's stage C and D; CP: clinical phase; CRC: colorectal cancer; PCDP: preclinical detectable phase; RCT: randomized controlled trial; TAMCAS: Taiwan Mulitcenter Cancer Screening

PCDP Dukes' CD compared with the transition rate from PCDP Dukes' AB to PCDP Dukes' CD was 1.41 (=0.2955/0.2095). The result of an RTR larger than 1 suggests that early detection of CRC plays a more important role in reducing the transition from PCDP Dukes' AB to PCDP Dukes' CD than in reducing the transition from PCDP Dukes' AB to CP Dukes' AB. The finding further suggests that selective screening with colonoscopy for this high-risk group is important for reducing advanced CRC (Dukes' CD), which in turn leads to a reduction in mortality from CRC. This indicator also corresponds to the effectiveness of the RCTs. Hardcastle et al. (1996) and Kronborg et al. (1996) showed a 15–18% reduction in CRC mortality with biennial gFOBT in two large population-based RCTs in Nottingham, UK and in Funen, Denmark. Chiu et al. (2011) made use of published data on the screening findings of these two trials and found that the RTR was 1.27 (=0.28/0.22).

As far as the reduction in the incidence of CRC is concerned, early detection of adenoma cannot be negligible. Yang et al. (2006) extended the previous five-state Markov model by inserting the adenoma stage as three states (diminutive, small, and large adenoma) into an eight-state Markov model and applied it to a community-based screening program with a fecal immunochemical test (FIT) in the Keelung community-based integrated screening (KCIS) in Taiwan. The incidence of diminutive adenoma in this general-risk population was 1.3 (95% CI: 1.0–1.6) per 1000. The researchers successfully estimated that the transition rates from diminutive to small adenoma, from small to large adenoma, and from large adenoma to preclinical adenoma were 0.0696 (95% CI: 0.0498–0.0895), 0.1854 (95% CI: 0.1163–0.2545), and 0.1772 (95% CI: 0.1099–0.2444), respectively.

9.3.2 The Nonhomogeneous Stochastic Processes

Wu et al. (2004) developed a computer algorithm to utilize the nonhomogeneous Markov process for modeling multistate disease progression. The simplest form of the Markov model assumed a time-homogeneous transition, namely, constant transition rates over time. However, this model always deviates from biological phenomena because the constant transition rate from disease-free to the PCDP considers that the incidence rate of preclinical cancer does not change with age. The Wu et al. method provided a flexible way to specify time homogeneous or nonhomogeneous (i.e., Weibull, and log-logistic distribution) Markov models. In Wong et al. (2004), the incidence of preclinical CRC was estimated to follow a Weibull distribution with a scale parameter of 1.45 per 100,000 and a shape parameter of 2.2824, which indicates an increasing trend of the incidence rate by age.

Not only is the age-dependent preclinical incidence of CRC considered but the sojourn time could also be time dependent. An alternative approach to dealing with the time nonhomogeneous multistate process is the semi-Markov model. Castelli et al. (2007) used this method to model the follow-up of patients with CRC undergoing curative resection. The multistate process involves three stages: alive without relapse (1), alive with relapse (2), and dead (3). The researchers were interested in the time-varying behavior of $1 \to 2$, $1 \to 3$, and $2 \to 3$. The constructed semi-Markov model was illustrated with the sojourn time of each transition following the Weibull distribution, although other distributions such as the gamma or log-normal distribution could be considered.

9.3.3 Heterogeneity Between Individuals

In addition to the nonhomogeneous transition rate issue, the transition rate could be individually different; for example, demographic characteristics of age and sex and clinical correlates might affect the transition rates. Hsieh et al. (2002) proposed a nonhomogeneous exponential regression Markov model to address this problem. The researchers used an exponential regression model to model the different characteristics of random processes between individuals. The consideration of relevant covariates in multistate transition models has implications for exploring the natural history of cancers. This can also accommodate the development of individually tailored screening.

The regression approach can also be used with the semi-Markov model when both time- and individual-dimension heterogeneity are considered. Castelli et al. (2007) incorporated patients' personal characteristics as covariates in the regression model for each transition to consider the effects of covariates on each transition.

9.4   Several Applications to Subsidiary Issues of Population-Based Screening for CRC

In this chapter, we also illustrate how the temporal disease natural history modeled by the underlying stochastic processes can be applied to different scenarios in relation to a series of subsidiary issues, including a case-cohort sampling design for elucidating the disease course of adenoma–carcinoma pathway for assessing the efficacy of reducing malignant transformation and the effectiveness of population-based screening programs, decision analysis, and its application with health economic decision models.

9.4.1   Case-cohort Design with Multistate Disease Process

The multistate model can be applied not only to the entire cohort from a population-based screening program but also to only a fraction of samples retrieved from hospital-based data or a cohort. Chen et al. (2003) used data from a case-cohort study to assess the natural history of adenoma-carcinoma and de novo carcinoma. In their study, they took random samples from three sets of patients with normal, polyp, and CRC findings. The Bayesian conversion was applied to construct the total likelihood for multistate Markov models (Chen et al. 2004) for the entire cohort who underwent colonoscopy in a medical center.

Their method provided an efficient way to elucidate the disease progress underpinning multistate disease progression. Furthermore, the stable convergence for parameter estimation with this Bayesian conversion enables the authors to account for one more parameter governing the transition directly from CRC-free to invasive CRC, so-called de novo carcinogenesis. Based on their estimated results with an incidence of diminutive adenoma of 0.0021 and of de novo CRC of 0.00095, they successfully quantified that approximately 32% of CRC cases arise from de novo sequences.

9.4.2   Efficacy of Reducing Malignant Transformation

The estimated natural history of the transition from premalignancy (adenoma) to invasive CRC can be used as the comparator for the observed transition of treated premalignancy to estimate the efficacy of reducing malignant transformation. In the Chen et al. (2003) hospital-series study, the ratio of the annual malignant transformation rate after polypectomy to progression from adenoma to cancer in light of natural history was 73% when the de novo pathway was taken into account. It is interesting to note that with consideration of the de novo pathway, the efficacy of polypectomy was greater (88%).

Cafferty et al. (2009) used a deterministic model to estimate the adenoma recurrence rate with data from follow-up colonoscopies in the National Polyp Study and the progression rate from adenoma to invasive cancers based on published data, from which an estimated reduction of between 97% and 99% in CRC incidence due to endoscopic surveillance in the National Polyp Study cohort was estimated.

9.4.3   Efficacy of population-based Screening by Various Screening Regimes

Elucidation of temporal disease natural history enables one in a straightforward way to estimate the effect of the inter-screening interval between screenings on mortality. Chen et al. (1999) estimated 26% (95% CI: 0–50%), 23% (95% CI: 0–48%), and 21% (95% CI: 0–47%) CRC mortality reductions for annual, biennial, and triennial screening regimes, respectively, for a selective screening program targeting at high-risk subjects with colonoscopy in combination with FOBT or double-contrast barium enema. However, such estimation was conservative because the benefit from early detection of adenoma was not taken into account.

Yang et al. (2006) found benefits of reducing mortality from CRC by 23% (3–40%), 15% (0–33%), and 11% (0–29%) for annual, biennial, and triennial screening regimes, respectively. This finding considered the benefit of treating adenoma. Note that in Yang et al. work, the screening modality was FIT with a program sensitivity of approximately 70%, which was inferior to that in TAMCAS in which the sensitivity for colonoscopy combined with FOBT was approximately 95%.

9.4.4 Decision Analysis of Population-based Screening for CRC

Understanding the disease's natural history is very helpful for building up a decision analysis for the evaluation of the effectiveness of population-based screening. The analytical decision analysis enables one to calculate sample size and statistical power before a large-scale population-based RCT can be designed and conducted. For example, Chiu et al. (2011) used a decision analysis model based on parameters for disease progression from two RCTs to calculate the required sample sizes, which were 86,150, and 65,592 subjects for the primary endpoint of mortality and the surrogate end point of advanced cancer rate, respectively, given a 70% attendance rate to the guaiac-FOBT screening and a 90% colonoscopy referral rate in a country with a 0.002 incidence of CRC in the target population aged 45–74 years.

9.4.5 Health Economic Decision Model

Economic evaluation of a population-based screening program is crucial for policy-makers, but it is a complex and multivariable problem. Cost-effectiveness analysis cannot be performed without a full assessment of the multistate process of disease using a modelling approach in order to assess the accumulated disease consequences and cost in each step based on different screening strategies, for example, inter-screening interval, starting and stopping age of screening, and cutoff value of FIT for referral for colonoscopy when the quantitative value is available. Chen et al. (2007) applied the estimated natural history of CRC from the KCIS by Yang et al. (2006) and determined the optimal cut-off of FIT by means of cost-effectiveness analysis. In their analysis, the screening program, irrespective of any cutoff value, dominated over no screening, namely, less cost and more effectiveness. However, the optimal cutoff was 110 ng/mL (OC-Sensor μ iFOBT kits, Eiken, Japan), which was determined as having the lowest incremental cost-effectiveness ratio.

9.4.6 Evaluation of Multiple Screening Modalities

In light of the many new technologies for the early detection of cancer, the application of multiple detection modalities in both opportunistic and population-based screening has increasingly gained attention. For example, in CRC screening, FOBT- and endoscopy-based screening modalities have been demonstrated to be effective in reducing mortality from CRC. One could use the stochastic process to elucidate the earliest times that an asymptomatic tumor can be detected by each screening tool. These findings can be used in modelling the disease natural history by dividing the preclinical screen-detectable phase (PCDP) of the disease into different epochs (Fig. 9.2). The proposed method can be flexibly applied to different

Fig. 9.2 Segmental sojourn times for multiple screening modalities with the targeted populations with different risk levels

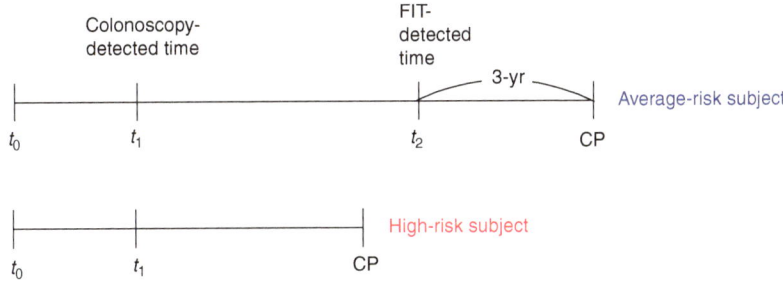

t_0: time for entering the PCDP
t_1: time for earliest detection with colonoscopy
t_2: time for earliest detection with FIT

scenarios of multiple screening tests used for the early diagnosis of cancer dispensing with assumptions regarding which test will be capable of detecting the tumor at the earliest time.

A mathematical modelling approach is an efficient alternative method for evaluating a series of subsidiary issues of population-based organized service screening dispensing with a randomized controlled trial study or a complex quasi-experimental study that requires the comparator. In conclusion, the multistate Markov model for the natural history of the disease can provide an indication of how fast the disease progresses and project the possible disease burden when no intervention is given. This method creates the opportunity to assess the treatment efficacy when a RCT is not feasible.

References

Cafferty FH, Sasieni PD, Duffy SW. A deterministic model for estimating the reduction in colorectal cancer incidence due to endoscopic surveillance. Stat Methods Med Res. 2009;18:163–82.

Castelli C, Combescure C, Foucher Y, Daures JP. Cost-effectiveness analysis in colorectal cancer using a semi-Markov model. Stat Med. 2007;26:5557–71.

Chiu HM, Chen SLS, Yen AMF, Chiu SYH, Fann JCY, Lee YC, et al. Effectiveness of fecal immunochemical testing in reducing colorectal cancer mortality from the One Million Taiwanese Screening Program. Cancer. 2015;121:3221–9.

Chen THH, Yen MF, Lai MS, Koong SL, Wang CY, Wong JM, Prevost TC, Duffy SW. Evaluation of a selective screening for colorectal carcinoma: the Taiwan Mulitcenter Cancer screening (TAMCAS) project. Cancer. 1999;86:1116–28.

Chen THH, Yen MF, Shiu MN, Tung TH, Wu HM. Stochastic model for non-standard case-cohort design. Stat Med. 2004;23:633–47.

Chen CD, Yen MF, Wang WM, Wong JM, Chen THH. A case-cohort study for the disease natural history of adenoma-carcinoma and de novo carcinoma and surveillance of colon and rectum after polypectomy: implication for efficacy of colonoscopy. Brit J Cancer. 2003;88:1866–73.

Chen LS, Liao CS, Chang SH, Lai HC, Chen THH. Cost-effectiveness analysis for determining optimal cut-off of immunochemical fecal occult blood test for population-based colorectal cancer screening (KCIS 16). J Med Screening. 2007;14(4):191–9.

Chen LS, Yen AM, Duffy SW, Tabar L, Lin WC, Chen HH. Computer-aided system of evaluation for population-based all-in-one service screening (CASE-PASS): from study design to outcome analysis with bias adjustment. Ann Epidemiol. 2010;20(10):786–96.

Chiu SY, Malila N, Yen AM, Anttila A, Hakama M, Chen HH. Analytical decision model for sample size and effectiveness projections for use in planning a population-based randomised controlled trial of colorectal cancer screening. J Eval Clin Pract. 2011;17:123–9.

Hardcastle JD, Chamberlain JO, Robinson MH, Moss SM, Amar SS, Balfour TW, et al. Randomised controlled trial of faecal-occult-blood screening for colorectal cancer. Lancet. 1996;348:1472–7.

Hsieh HJ, Chen THH, Chang SH. Assessing chronic disease progression using non-homogenous exponential regression Markov models. Stat Med. 2002;21:3369–82.

Kronborg O, Fenger C, Olsen J, Jorgensen OD, Sondergaard O. Randomised study of screening for colorectal cancer with faecal-occult-blood test. Lancet. 1996;348:1467–71.

Mandel JS, Bond JH, Church TR, Snover DC, Bradley GM, Schuman LM, et al. Reducing mortality from colorectal cancer by screening for fecal occult blood. Minnesota Colon Cancer Control Study N Engl J Med. 1993;328:1365–71.

Wong JM, Yen MF, Lai MS, Duffy SW, Smith RA, Chen THH. Progression rates of colorectal cancer by dukes' stage in a high-risk group: analysis of selective colorectal cancer screening. Cancer J. 2004;10:160–9.

Wu HM, Yen MF, Chen THH. SAS macro program for non-homogeneous Markov process in modeling multi-state disease progression. Comput Methods Prog Biomed. 2004;75:95–105.

Yang KC, Liao CS, Chiu YH, Yen MF, Chen THH. Colorectal cancer screening with fecal occult blood test within a multiple disease screening program: an experience from Keelung, Taiwan. J Med Screen. 2006;13(Suppl 1):8–13.

Cost-Effectiveness Analysis of Colorectal Cancer Screening

Jean Ching-Yuan Fann, Abbie Ting-Yu Lin,
Rene Wei-Jung Chang, and Hsiu-Hsi Chen

Abstract

While the efficacy of population-based screening for colorectal cancer (CRC) with the fecal occult blood test (FOBT) has been demonstrated in several randomized controlled trials the results on cost-effectiveness analysis using a probabilistic approach has been barely investigated. In this chapter, we first proposed the framework of economic evaluation for population-based screening for CRC and then reviewed the results in literature on various screening methods. We also demonstrate a case study with the application of the analytical Markov decision model to evaluating different screening strategies with particular emphasis on fecal immunochemical test (FIT) that has been implemented in Taiwan since 2000. The probabilistic cost-effectiveness analysis was performed to evaluate annual, biennial, and triennial FIT as opposed to no screening. We found biennial FIT was cost saving compared with the annual g-FOBT test. The probability of being cost-effective was up to 80% given 20,000 WTP. Performing cost-effective analysis with a probabilistic approach plays a crucial in evidence-based medicine for population-based screening policy.

Keywords

Economic evaluation · Fecal immunochemical test · Guaiac–fecal blood occult test Inter-screening interval · Screening

10.1 Economic Evaluation of Population-Based Cancer Screening

From the viewpoint of economics, population-based screening has pros and cons. The greatest merit of population-based screening is the ability to reduce a large proportion of deaths from colorectal cancer (CRC) through early detection and to potentially reduce the incidence of CRC through the removal of advanced adenoma. However, the benefit accrued from screening occurs later than the cost incurred at the inception of screening. This aspect is more crucial in determining costs for the comparison of the screened group with the unscreened group, particularly when there is a long disease natural history of

J. C.-Y. Fann (✉)
Department of Health Industry Management, College of Healthcare Management, Kainan University, Taoyuan, Taiwan
e-mail: jeanfann@mail.knu.edu.tw

A. T.-Y. Lin · R. W.-J. Chang · H.-H. Chen
Institute of Epidemiology and Preventive Medicine, College of Public Health, National Taiwan University, Taipei, Taiwan
e-mail: chenlin@ntu.edu.tw

© Springer Nature Singapore Pte Ltd. 2021
H.-M. Chiu, H.-H. Chen (eds.), *Colorectal Cancer Screening*,
https://doi.org/10.1007/978-981-15-7482-5_10

colorectal neoplasms. Neglecting such a time preference reflected in time-stamped disease natural history between the two groups may lead to a biased result of cost-effectiveness/utility analysis and cost-benefit analysis.

10.1.1 Factors Affecting the Effectiveness of Colorectal Cancer Screening

The effectiveness of CRC screening is highly dependent on a host of factors, including the disease's natural history as mentioned in Chap. 9, screening modalities, attendance rate for screening participation, compliance rate with the referrals for abnormal findings, provided treatment, and cumulative survival after diagnosis. The natural history of the disease plays an important role in the early detection of asymptomatic CRC as noted in Chap. 9. The longer the duration of asymptomatic phases, the earlier the disease is likely to be detected. Early-detected CRCs resulting from screening can result in the advance of the date of diagnosis, so-called lead time, in comparison with those in the absence of screening, and, in turn, prolonged survival if the lead time is gained before the curable time point. The second factor related to the effectiveness of screening is the attendance rate for screening participation. It is evident that the high effectiveness in terms of mortality reduction is determined by a high attendance rate. It is interesting to note that a low attendance rate not only leads to lower effectiveness but also invokes enormous costs attributed to later treatment in the absence of screening. The rate of compliance with the referral process also has a large influence on the effectiveness of screening. A typical example is demonstrated in population-based CRC screening with the fecal occult blood test (FOBT) or fecal immunochemical test (FIT). The effectiveness is reduced if the compliance rate with the colonoscopy offered to screenees with FOBT or FIT positivity is poor. Cumulative survival associated with early detection is also pivotal in the effectiveness of screening. Cumulative survival is affected by several features, including therapeutic components and

treatment modality. The natural history of the disease may vary by racial or ethnic groups. Organization features such as attendance rate and referral rate also vary from country to country. Dimensions or perspectives of cost incurred from screening or treatment are affected by the consumer price index, utilization rates of medical consultation, and economic scale, which also vary across countries.

10.1.2 Cost Considerations in Population-Based Organized Service Screening

Costs incurred as a result of population-based screening are very complex. The cost in the initial screening stage is tremendous because of initial investment in manpower, facility, and consumables. It is hoped that the reduction in advanced disease as a result of screening will reduce expenditure associated with treatment costs. In addition, the concept of cost in economic analysis not only implies true expenditure but is also valued as an opportunity cost for the value of all alternative uses of the expenditure.

According to Weinstein and Finberg (1980), the cost involved in the production of a good or a service is denoted by production costs. Production cost can be deconstructed into three components: direct cost, overhead cost, and induced cost. Direct costs include the cost of material, equipment, and labor (professional or nonprofessional). Overhead cost represents the costs of all other items related to health and medical care services for screening, including space and administration services. Induced costs are symbolic of costs that are caused by service screening that would not have been incurred in the absence of the screening. These included costs related to false-positive cases and increased costs associated with continuing to treat screenees who live longer because of the service screening. Indirect cost is related to the cost of lost productivity and monetary values. Economic assessment assesses whether and how the benefit of screening in terms of reducing advanced disease or death can outweigh the cost incurred in the initial screening.

10.1.3 Framework of the Economic Evaluation of Population-Based CRC Screening

Figure 10.1 shows the overall structure of the economic evaluation of population-based CRC screening from the invitation of screenees in the population registry, the disease natural history, and the identification of true-positive cases, false-positive cases, false-negative cases, and true-negative cases, which depends on the performance of screening tools. True-negative cases may be associated with induced negative costs due to reassurance of true-negative status, which in turn, increases production. False-positive cases may lead to induced positive costs because of the costs involved in referral and confirmatory processes. False-negative cases increase treatment costs associated with advanced diseases. Prevalent/incident cases become involved with early treatment costs and probably augment costs as suggested above. In addition to direct costs, indirect costs related to production loss resulting from the service screening or delayed treatment must be considered.

Each case diagnosed between screens (interval cancer) or detected by the screening (prevalent screen or incident screen) can be dealt with using different approaches with different costs. Non-attenders often have delayed treatment and die early. Patients with interval cancers may have delayed treatment. Both may have costs associated with terminal care. Outcome measurements for effectiveness are advanced cancer, subsequent complications or disability, death, and life expectancy.

10.1.4 Formal Economic Analysis

To balance costs and effectiveness, formal economic analysis should be conducted. Methods of economic evaluation include cost-effectiveness/utility analysis and cost-benefit analysis. Cost-effectiveness/utility analysis is used to choose the most economical strategy among all possible choices. Cost-benefit analysis is employed to assess whether the intervention program is worthwhile or how much additional benefit can be produced by the intervention program. In cost-benefit

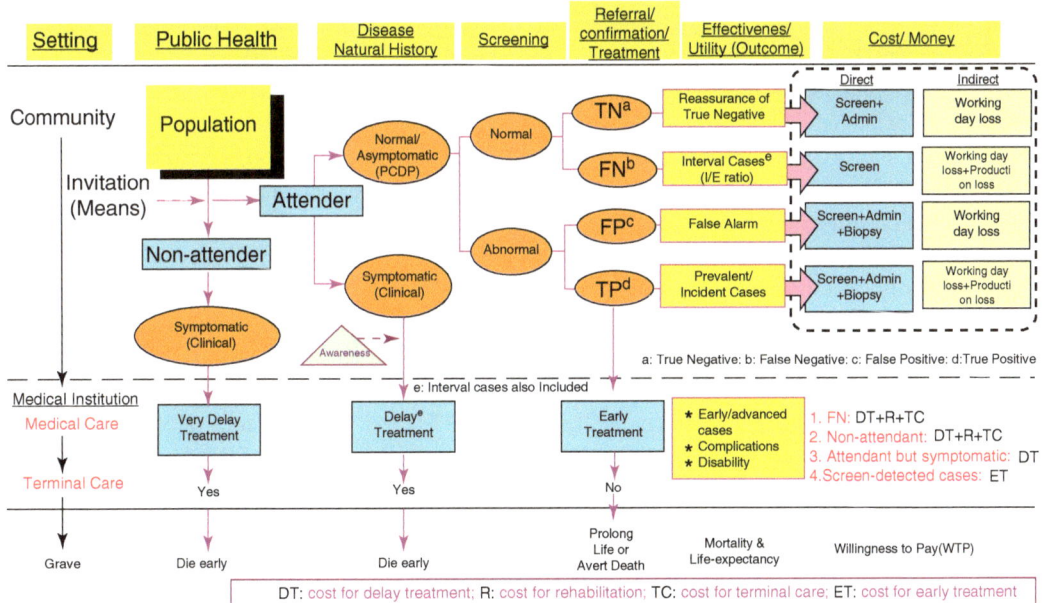

Fig. 10.1 Framework of economic evaluation of population-based CRC screening

analysis, effectiveness is translated into benefit in terms of human capital approach or willingness to pay (WTP).

10.2 Current Evidence on Cost-Effectiveness Analysis of Colorectal Cancer Screening

There have been numerous studies addressing the cost-effectiveness of CRC screening using a variety of screening modalities, including guaiac-FOBT (gFOBT), FIT, colonoscopy, and flexible sigmoidoscopy. Table 10.1 lists the detailed results in terms of cost and effectiveness. We extracted the data on incremental cost and incremental effectiveness of the methods targeting the general population aged 50–69 years from these studies and plotted the results shown on the incremental cost-effectiveness plane (incremental CE plane) for the comparisons of annual gFOBT (Fig. 10.2a), annual FIT (Fig. 10.2b), biennial FIT (Fig. 10.2c), colonoscopy (Fig. 10.2d), and flexible sigmoidoscopy (FS) (Fig. 10.2e) with no screening. Although the comparison between these studies from different countries could be affected by other features, such as disease burden, ethnic group, level of medical expenditure, cost of screening and referral modalities, and compliance with regular screening and referral, we can still identify a pattern of cost-effectiveness of CRC screening based on screening modalities. Because the cost of stool-based screening is low, the incremental cost-effectiveness ratio (ICER) of the majority of stool-based screening is below $20,000. However, a trend toward better effectiveness was observed for annual FIT, followed by biennial FIT and gFOBT. For annual FIT, many studies show cost-saving results (the fourth quadrant in the incremental CE plane (Fig. 10.2b). Generally, colonoscopy can be the most effective among all these screening modalities (Fig. 10.2d), whereas annual FIT could achieve similar results in terms of effectiveness but at a lower cost (Fig. 10.2b).

10.3 A Case Study of a Cost-Effectiveness Analysis of Colorectal Cancer Screening with Fecal Immunochemical Test (FIT) in Taiwan

The burden of morbidity and mortality attributed to CRC has been seen not only in developed countries but also in developing countries with high economic development, such as Taiwan. In 2016, CRC was ranked as the second most common cancer. The age-standardized incidence and mortality rates were 41.29 and 14.45 per 100,000, respectively.

gFOBT was widely used as a CRC screening tool because of its feasibility, and its efficacy has been proven by randomized control trials (Mandel et al. 1993; Kronborg et al. 1996; Hardcastle et al. 1996). However, gFOBT has been criticized for its low sensitivity. Several kinds of gFOBTs have been developed in past decades. Their availability and performance are quite different. The FIT is highly recommended because it has a balance between sensitivity and specificity, has higher sensitivity for advanced adenoma and early-stage cancers, and it can achieve higher compliance without dietary or drug restriction. However, its price was two- to five-fold that of gFOBT (Young et al. 2002).

The inter-screening interval of gFOBT has been traditionally recommended for 1 year. Since FIT is more capable of detecting CRC than gFOBT with an acceptable specificity and a higher cost, the debate is ongoing if the inter-screening interval could be lengthened to 2 years or longer. In fact, there are many countries that have provided biennial gFOBT or FIT for CRC screening (Benson et al. 2008). However, there are still rare studies evaluating the cost-effectiveness of CRC screening by FIT with a screening interval longer than 1 year compared with annual gFOBT screening in countries with a low-to-medium incidence of CRC.

We performed a probabilistic cost-effectiveness analysis with a Markov decision model to compare annual, biennial, and 3-yearly FIT screening with no screening targeting an

Fig. 10.2 Cost-effectiveness analysis for colorectal cancer screening with various kinds of screening modality versus no screen (**a**) annual gFOBT vs no screen (**b**) annual FIT vs no screen (**c**) biennal FIT vs no screen (**d**) colonoscopy vs no screen (**e**) flexible sigmoidoscopy vs no screen

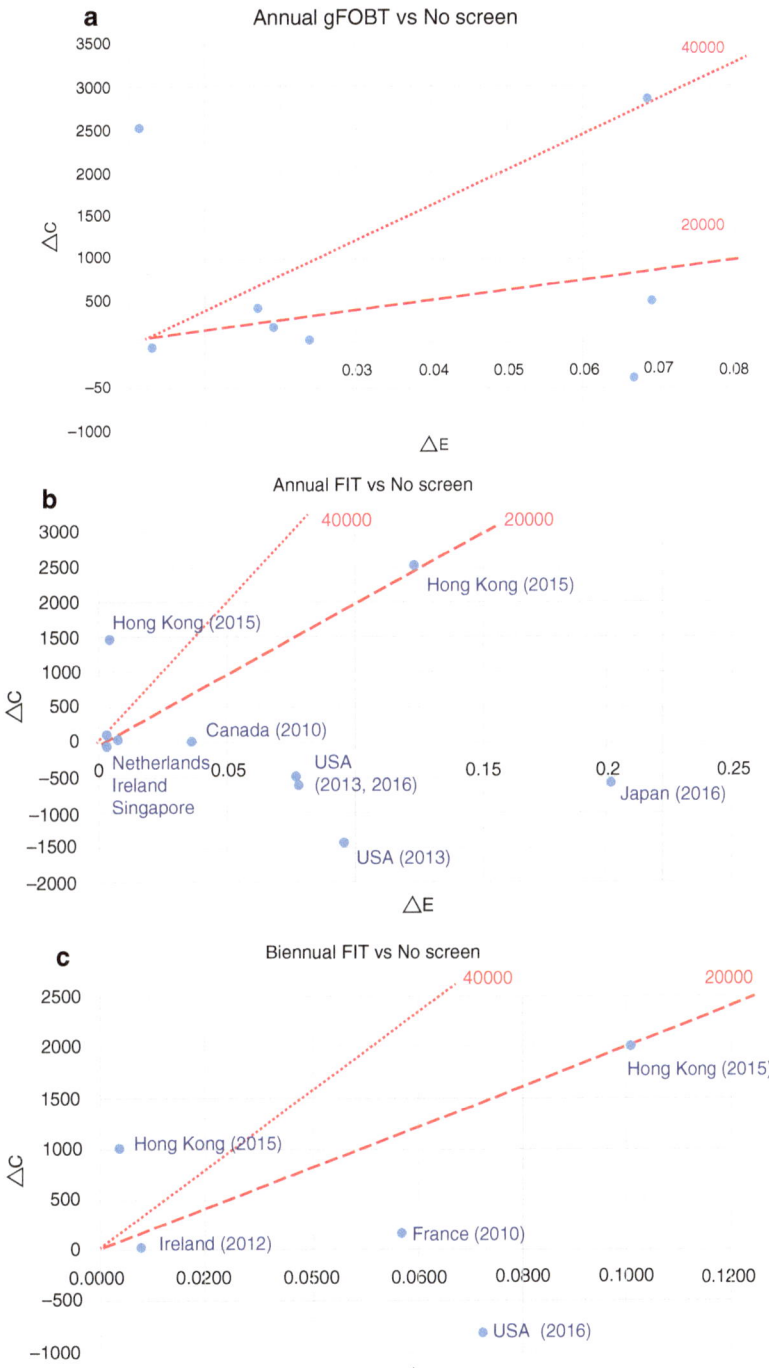

Fig. 10.2 (continued)

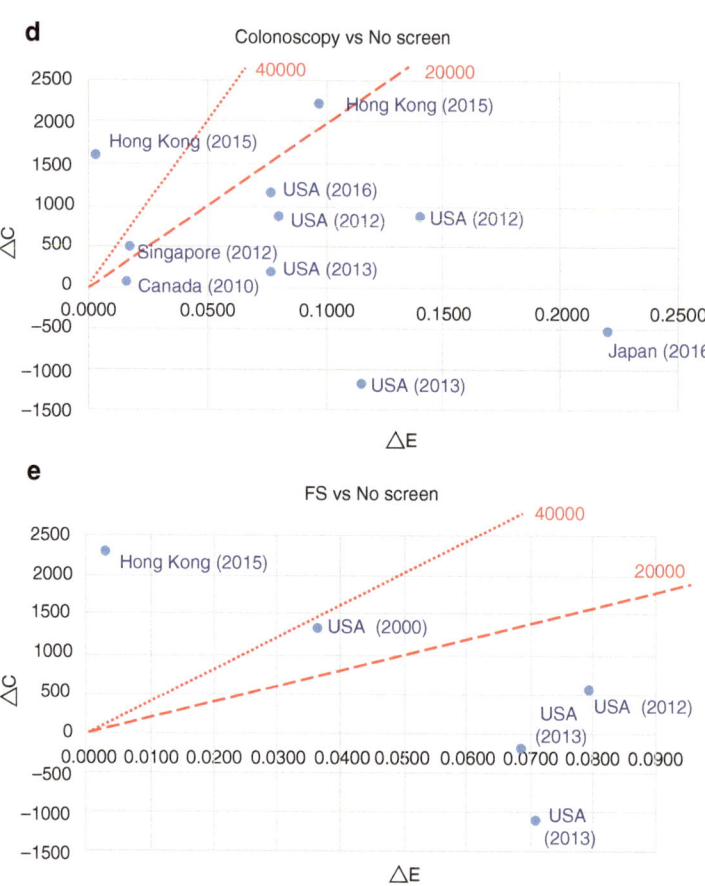

average-risk population from the perspective of the health administrative body.

10.4 Empirical Community-Based Screening Data

10.4.1 Screened Population

We used empirical data to estimate the proportions of demographic subgroups, attendance rates, and referral rates from the Keelung Community-based Integrated Screening (KCIS) program, which included screening for CRC, four other neoplastic diseases and three nonneoplastic chronic diseases since 1999. FIT screening in KCIS is actually the pilot study of the current FIT–based Taiwan CRC Screening Program. The detailed study design and preliminary results of the KCIS program

were described in full elsewhere (Chen et al. 2004).

Community-based CRC screening with FIT was utilized in the KCIS program. This program was implemented in 1999 and continued till the launch of the national program in 2004. The high identification of asymptomatic cases, the enhancement of the attendance rate for Pap smear screening for cervical cancer, and the efficiency of follow-up have been demonstrated (Chen et al. 2004). The target population consisted of KCIS attendees aged 50–79 years between 1999 and 2004 after excluding those who had previous CRC, genetic disorders such as familial adenomatous polyposis, or hereditary nonpolyposis. Finally, the total population consisted of 32,201 KCIS attendees aged 50–79 years old in the first year they were invited for FIT between 1999 and 2004.

10.4.2 Screening Protocol and Referrals

In each outreach and on-site screening scenario of the KCIS program, we offered the FIT tube for participants. Each attendant was also taught via an illustration in a pamphlet how stool samples were collected. The kit was returned to collection centers within 3–5 days. After testing, subjects with positive findings were arranged to undergo colonoscopy. The referral system in the KCIS program provided a door-to-door service for sending subjects with positive FIT results to designated hospitals. Polyps were removed by polypectomy, and a biopsy was sent to confirm malignancy status. Information on adenoma size and histological type of polyps was also collected.

10.4.3 Cost-Effectiveness Analysis with the Markov Decision Model

10.4.3.1 The Disease Natural History of CRC

We referred to an eight-state Markov model developed by Yang et al. (2006) as reviewed in Chap. 9. We also used the transition rates estimated by that study. We then used those transition rates and annual age- and sex-specific mortality rates of all causes from the life table to estimate the age- and sex-specific transition probabilities in 1 year.

10.4.3.2 Analytical Markov Decision Model

A Markov decision model was built to predict cost, life years gained (LYG), and other outcomes of interest. We combined the diminutive adenoma and small adenoma states into the same state referred to as "small adenoma" in the decision tree. The basic assumption of such a Markov model is based on the Markov memoryless property, so the transition probability P_{ij} for one individual going into state j from state i depends on current state i, regardless of the pathway through which the individual went. Each cycle is 1 year. Figure 10.3a shows the first two parts of the decision tree. The first part after the decision node includes screening strategies, covering no screening, annual guaiac-FOBT (denoted by gFOBT1), and FIT (OC-Sensor) with one- to three-year screening intervals (denoted by FIT1, FIT2, FIT3, respectively).

The second part after each strategy mentioned above is the possible states, including all the states of natural history and the conditions of follow-up. The probabilities under each Markov state are the initial probabilities at the start of the Markov cycle. Because we targeted the asymptomatic population, the distribution of initial probabilities was therefore the prevalence of each state when entering the screening program. The Dirichlet distribution was used for initial probabilities estimated from empirical data of the KCIS program (Table 10.1).

The third part is shown in Fig. 10.3b. Those states after each initial state were transition states, and the probabilities under each branch are the transition probabilities in one cycle. We used one subtree (small adenoma) to illustrate the process of screening. If the invitee had continuous compliance with CRC screening (the probability was denoted by p_cont), then he/she would complete this screen, and the screening cost would be incurred currently. The probability of having a positive test depended on the sensitivity (sen_FIT_sa: the sensitivity of FIT for small adenoma). On the other hand, if the attendee was in a normal state, the probability of being negative was the specificity.

The further consequences after screening but before treatment would be guided by referral rate (denoted by p_ref), perforation rate (denoted by p_perfor), and perforation death rate (denoted by p_perford). The later consequences and the corresponding cost were determined. We used the beta distribution to model the probabilities of those situations with binary outcomes under conditions of uncertainty (Table 10.1).

As far as the treatment process is concerned, we calculated the medical cost during the first 4 years after diagnosis. Since the distribution of medical cost is usually positively skewed, log-transformation was used to improve the normality. Therefore, we used the log-normal distribution

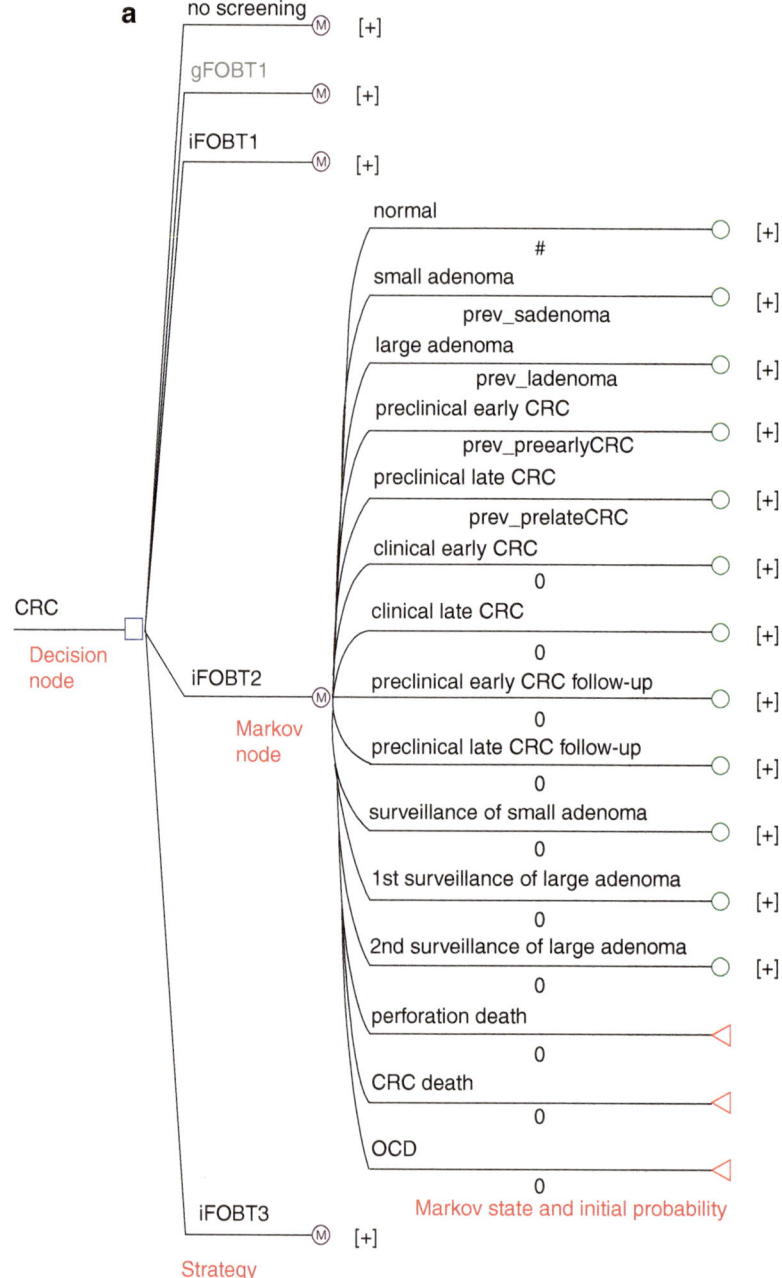

Fig. 10.3 (**a**) Structure of the Markov model. (**b**) Structure of subtree: taking small adenoma as an example

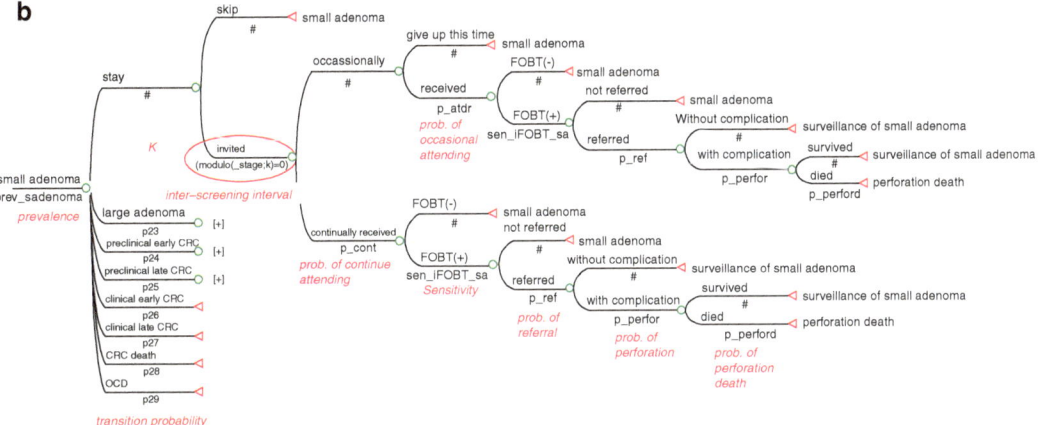

Fig. 10.3 (continued)

to model medical cost by stage of CRC (Table 10.1). However, not all cost items could be estimated from KCIS data, so we referred to the local studies that had investigated the related cost.

The surveillance process with one colonoscopy in the fourth year after polypectomy for small adenoma and large adenoma and the ninth year after polypectomy for large adenoma was also embedded in the decision model. If some screen-detected cases with adenoma had gone through the surveillance process and remained normal, then he/she returned to the routine screening program.

10.4.3.3 Computer Simulation

The starting age and sex of the hypothetical cohort were simulated with the makeup of demographic features identical to the same age-sex distribution of invitees for CRC screening from KCIS attendees. We classified six subgroups by sex and age groups. The starting age was the middle age of each group, i.e., the three starting ages were 55, 65, and 75 years. The end point was the year of death or the age of 80 years old whichever came first. We used the life-years gained as the outcome of effectiveness.

The results are presented as incremental cost-effectiveness ratios (ICER) and acceptability curves. We used "Willingness to Pay" (WTP)

(Briggs et al. 2002) as the threshold to accept the additional cost paid for one life-year gained. We took USD$20,000 as the base case of WTP in the model, which was around the GDP per capita in Taiwan in 2012, and we also plotted acceptability curves based on a range of WTP from $0 to $40,000.

Some parameters were assumed arbitrarily. One of them is the discount rate, assigned as 3%, which has been suggested by the US panel. Both cost and LYG were discounted at the same discount rate. Table 10.1 shows the point estimate or distribution of parameters.

10.4.3.4 Key Assumptions

- The transition probabilities were homogeneous within the subgroup of the same sex and age group.
- The treatment efficacy depended on the stage of CRC; hence, the survival rate was only dependent on stage.
- The recurrence rate of adenoma was ignored. We assumed that the incidence rates of adenoma between normal people and those who had been treated were equal.
- The medical expenditure from the first 4 years and the year of death accounted for almost all medical expenditures after the year of CRC diagnosis.

Table 10.1 Base case values or distributions of parameters

Variable	Base-case values	Range or distribution	References
I. The disease natural history and prognosis			
Prevalence of initial state (normal; small adenoma; small adenoma; preclinical early CRC; preclinical late CRC)			KCIS (2000–2004); Wu et al. (2006)
Aged 55 years, male		Dirichlet (4032,536,248,8,5)	
Aged 55 years, female		Dirichlet (8125,1081,499,16,11)	
Aged 65 years, male		Dirichlet (3310,543,275,9,6)	
Aged 65 years, female		Dirichlet (5029,826,418,14,9)	
Aged 75 years, male		Dirichlet (2044,517,299,10,7)	
Aged 75 years, female		Dirichlet (2141,541,314,10,7)	
Annual transition rate			
Normal → diminutive adenoma	0.0013	Gamma (72,55490)	Yang et al. (2006)
Diminutive → small adenoma	0.0696	Gamma (47,675)	Yang et al. (2006)
Small → large adenoma	0.1854	Gamma (27.6,149)	Yang et al. (2006)
Large adenoma → preclinical early CRC	0.1772	Gamma (26.6,150)	Yang et al. (2006)
Preclinical early → preclinical late CRC	0.3079	Gamma (16, 52)	Yang et al. (2006)
Preclinical early → clinical early CRC	0.2455	Gamma (14.7, 60)	Yang et al. (2006)
Preclinical late → clinical late CRC	0.9241	Gamma (7.3, 7.9)	Yang et al. (2006)
Early CRC (dukes' A&B) → death	0.0299	Gamma (9.9,330)	NTUH data
Late CRC (dukes' C&D) → death	0.1526	Gamma (71.4,468)	NTUH data
Annual mortality associated with all-cause death by age			Life Table (2002)
III. Test characteristics			
Sensitivity			
For small adenoma (<10 mm)			
gFOBT	0.028	Beta (3,106)	Greenberg et al. (2000)
FIT	0.102	Beta (62,548)	Cheng et al. (2002)
For large adenoma (> = 10 mm)			
gFOBT	0.205	Beta (8,31)	Greenberg et al. (2000)
FIT	0.515	Beta (86,81)	Cheng et al. (2002), Levi et al. (2007)
For CRC			
gFOBT	0.510	Beta (25,24)	Allison et al. (1996), Greenberg et al. (2000)
FIT	0.827	Beta (67,14)	Cheng et al. (2002), Chen et al. (2007), Levi et al. (2007)
Specificity			
gFOBT	0.981	Beta (7771,152)	Allison et al. (1996)
FIT	0.939	Beta (28,421,1861)	Cheng et al. (2002), Chen et al. (2007), Levi et al. (2007)
IV. Screening characteristics			
Compliance (proportions of different compliance behaviors in terms of undergoing FOBT among KCIS)			
Attendees(continually; occasionally)	0.796	Beta (10171,2614)	KCIS (2000–2004)

Table 10.1 (continued)

Variable	Base-case values	Range or distribution	References
Attendance rate for those undergoing FOBT occasionally	0.407	Beta (2169,3160)	KCIS (2000–2004)
Referral rate	0.714	Beta (2811,1125)	KCIS (2000–2004)
Complication of colonoscopy			
Severe complication rate	0.003	Beta (162,57580)	Whitlock et al. (2008)
Death rate due to perforation	0.00001	Beta (1,9999)#	Wu et al. (2006)
V. Unit cost, USD			
Screening cost			
gFOBT	0.7		NHIA
FIT	4		NHIA
Confirmation cost			
Colonoscopy for diagnosis only	68		NHIA
Colonoscopy combined with polypectomy	181		NHIA
Treatment cost			
For preclinical early CRC			
1st year	215	Lognormal (3.6847, 3.3671)	KCIS (2000–2004)
2nd year	41	Lognormal (2.5044, 2.4324)	
3rd year	20	Lognormal (2.1551, 1.6359)	
4th year	15	Lognormal (1.7302, 1.9655)	
For preclinical late CRC			
1st year	1912	Lognormal (5.7877, 3.536)	KCIS (2000–2004)
2nd year	439	Lognormal (4.6554, 2.8595)	
3rd year	1201	Lognormal (6.0279, 2.1265)	
4th year	410	Lognormal (4.9020, 2.2302)	
For clinical CRC			
1st year	4003	Lognormal (6.5779, 3.4337)	KCIS (2000–2004)
2nd year	2451	Lognormal (6.5033, 2.6017)	
3rd year	257	Lognormal (4.0948, 2.2902)	
4th year	1546	Lognormal (5.9731, 2.7402)	
For terminal care due to CRC	9455	Uniform (7879,11031)[b]	Wu et al. (2006), Chen et al. (2007)
For complication cost of perforation	1667		Wu et al. (2006)
For complication cost of perforation death	2818		Wu et al. (2006)
VI. Discount rate	0.03		

Abbreviations: *CRC* colorectal cancer, *KCIS* Keelung Community Integrated Screening, *NHIA* National Health Insurance Administration, *NTUH* National Taiwan University Hospital

[a]The estimates were re-estimated from data resources

[b]The point estimates were derived from data resources and assigned a conservative prior distribution for probabilistic sensitivity analysis

10.5 Results

10.5.1 FIT Screening by Inter-Screening Interval

Table 10.2 shows the mean, standard deviation, median, and 2.5% and 97.5% percentiles (as 95% CI) of cost and effectiveness of the 300 samples

with a sample size of 10000 based on the probabilistic approach. We also calculated the ICER using the mean value of cost and LYG associated with different strategies. The results show that all screening strategies were cost saving when compared with "no screening." Compared with gFOBT1, FIT1 and FIT2 were cost saving and FIT3 was cost-effective.

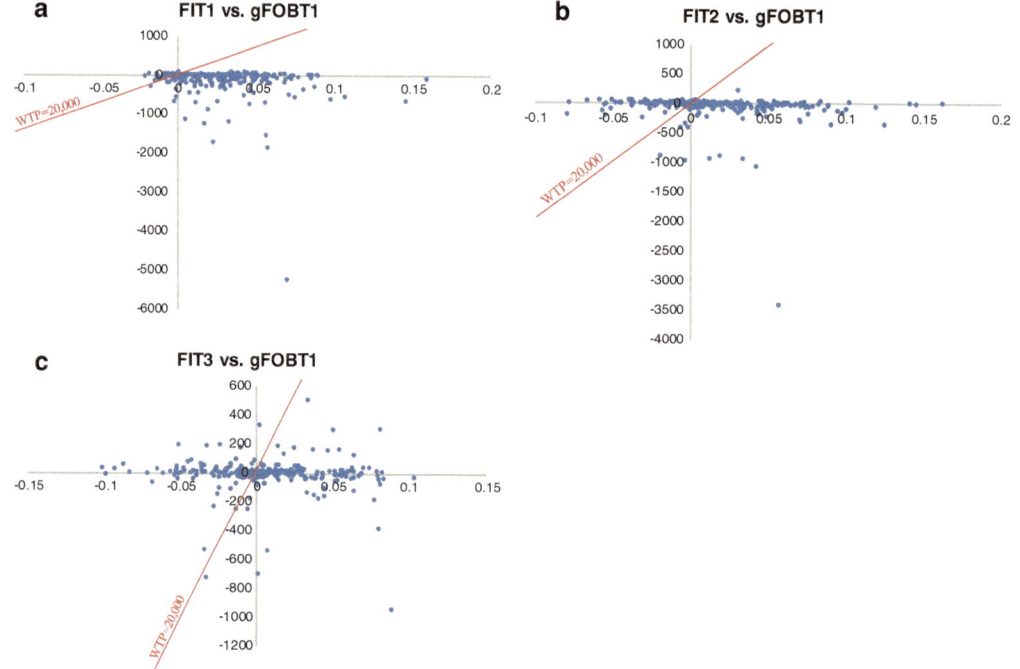

Fig. 10.4 (**a**) Incremental cost-effectiveness scatter plot (FIT1 vs. gFOBT1). (**b**) Incremental cost-effectiveness scatter plot (FIT2 vs. gFOBT1). (**c**) Incremental cost-effectiveness scatter plot (FIT3 vs. gFOBT1)

Table 10.2 The results of cost and life-years gained associated with different CRC screening strategies by using a probabilistic decision analysis

Strategy	Cost, $ Mean (2.5%, 97.5%)	Life-years gained (LYG) Mean (2.5%, 97.5%)	ICER[1] ($/LYG)	ICER[2] ($/LYG)
No screening	1257 (250, 5628)	12.713 (12.628,12.798)	Reference	–
gFOBT1	684 (136,3063)	12.762 (12.675,12.844)	−11,784	Reference
FIT3	685 (140,3385)	12.770 (12.687,12.847)	−10,101	125
FIT2	592 (144,2755)	12.782 (12.700,12.858)	−9690	−4600
FIT1	468 (159,1839)	12.802 (12.724,12.878)	−8902	−5400

ICER[1]: Treating no screening as the reference group
ICER[2]: Treating gFOBT1 as the reference group

Figure 10.4 shows the probabilities of FIT with different inter-screening intervals being cost-effective when compared with gFOBT1. The results show that both FIT1 had 79% probabilities of being cost-effective based on a WTP of $20,000 per LYG. The corresponding figures for FIT2 and FIT3 were 66% and 57%, respectively.

10.6 Discussion

In spite of a series of randomized controlled trials that have demonstrated the effectiveness of population-based screening for CRC, health policy-makers are often faced with whether the gain from the effectiveness of reducing mortality and advanced stage CRC can outweigh the costs involved in such a large-scale screening program in terms of cost-effectiveness analysis, one of the criteria for evidence-based medicine. In this chapter, we demonstrated a cost-effectiveness analysis with empirical data on FIT screening derived from a community-based screening program in Keelung, a northern city of Taiwan. When we used annual gFOBT as the reference group, both FIT1 and FIT2 are cost saving. This means that the inter-screening interval of FIT could be lengthened to 2 years. The reason annual FIT is the best and most cost-saving strategy is that its cost input in the initial stage of the screening program could be compensated by the reduction in cost input for CRC treatment. However, even if the total cost is saved, the constraint of the initial cost input still exists, and the clinical capacity is also limited. Therefore, if a country or a local government could not provide resources to input during the initial period of the CRC screening program, biennial FIT may be a suitable strategy.

The method used for cost-effectiveness analysis here is not based on a randomized controlled design but resorts to a Markov decision model that was constructed to capture the disease natural history of CRC in the light of a modelling approach mentioned in Chap. 9 to simulate the control group in the absence of screening. Other screening strategies following the analytical Markov decision model on the disease natural history were evaluated by inserting the parameters related to basic screening characteristics such as attendance rate, sensitivity and specificity of the screening tool, and the referral rate to give the yields of primary end point for each screening strategy. The probability approach was used to model the probability of being cost-effective with the simulated Monte Carlo plane and the acceptability curve. The main reason of using analytical Markov decision model rather than a randomized controlled trial is to model the mechanism from the input of screening strategies to the output of primary outcomes in order to capture the uncertainty of influential parameters affecting the 95% ICER values and the probability of being cost-effective using the probabilistic approach.

In conclusion, we demonstrated a probabilistic cost-effectiveness analysis with parameters derived from the pilot study of Taiwanese program and found that FIT screening compared with no screening was cost saving. Lengthening the inter-screening interval to 2 years for CRC screening with FIT was still cost saving compared to the costs associated with annual gFOBT.

Supplementary Table 10.1
Literatures of Cost-Effectiveness
Analysis for Colorectal Cancer

Country/Author/Year	Target population	Strategies	Outcome measures/results
Australia Salkeld et al. (1996)	Participants 50–80 years of age in the Minnesota RCT	(I) Annual FOBT (II) No screen	ICER (I)/(II): AUD 24,660/LYS
US Sonnenberg et al. (2000)	50 years of age in the general population	(I) Annual FOBT (II) sigmoidoscopy every 5 years (III) Colonoscopy every 5 years (IV) No screen	ICER (I)/(IV): USD 9705/LYS (II)/(IV): USD 36,509/LYS (III)/(IV): USD 10,983/LYS (II)/(I): USD 65,704/LYS (III)/(I): USD 11,382/LYS (III)/(II): Dominant
US Frazier et al. (2000)	50-years of age US population at average risk of CRC	(I) Rehydrated FOBT (II) Unrehydrated FOBT (III) sigmoidoscopy (IV) DCBE (V) Colonoscopy (VI) No screen	Compliance is assumed to be 60% with the initial screen and 80% with follow-up or surveillance colonoscopy. ICER (II) + (III) every 10 years/(III) every 10 years: USD 21,200/LYS (II) + (III) every 5 years/(II) + (III) every 5 years: USD 51,200/LYS (I) + (III) every 5 years/(II) + (III) every 5 years: USD 92,900/LYS
US Ladabaum et al. (2001)	50–80 years of age with no specific risks for colon cancer	(I) Aspirin chemoprophylaxis (II) FS every 5 years and annual FOBT (III) colonoscopy every 10 years (IV) no screen	ICER (I)/(IV): Dominant (II)/(IV): USD 16,844/LYS (III)/(IV): USD 20,172/LYS (I) + (II)/(I): USD 26,315/LYS (I) + (III)/(I): USD 30,822/LYS (I) + (II)/(II): Dominated (I) + (III)/(III): USD 149,161/LYS
US McMahon et al. (2001)	Average-risk populations	(I) Annual FOBT(II) biennial FOBT (III) FS(IV) colonoscopy (V) DCBE	ICER (V) every 3 years or (V) every 5 years + (I) compared with next cheapest strategy: ICER < USD 55,600/LYS (V) every 3 years + (I) compared with next cheapest strategy: ICER > USD 100,000/LYS (IV) compared with next cheapest strategy: ICER > USD 100,000/LYS
US Suleiman et al. (2002)	50 years of age in the general population	(I) Colonoscopy once per 10 years and every 3 years in subjects with polyps(II) chemoprevention with 325 mg of daily aspirin(III) no screen	ICER (I)/(III): USD 10,983/LYS(II)/(III): USD 47,249/LYS(I) + (II)/(III): USD 41,929/LYS(I) + (II)/(I): USD 227,607/LYS(I) + (II)/(II): USD 34,836/LYS

Country/Author/ Year	Target population	Strategies	Outcome measures/results
US van Ballegooijen et al. (2003)	People who have never been screened before 65 years of age and who use FOBT as the only method of screening after 65 years of age.	(I) gFOBT (Hemoccult II, Sensa)(II) FIT	ICER *If a specificity of 98% for iFOBT,* (II)/(I, Hemoccult II): • Dominant (A unit cost of $4.5 for both tests). • $11,000/LYS (A unit cost of $28 for (II), and a unit of cost of $4.5 for (I, Hemoccult II)) (II)/(I, Sensa): Dominant *If a specificity of 95% for iFOBT,* (II)/(I, Hemoccult II): • $6000/LYS (A unit cost of $4.5 for both tests) • $21,000/LYS (A unit cost of $28 for (II), and a unit of cost of $4.5 for (I, Hemoccult II)). (II)/(I, Sensa): • Dominant (A unit cost of $4.5 for both tests). $8,517,000/LYS(A unit cost of $28 for (II), and a unit of cost of $4.5 for (I, Hemoccult II))
France Berchi et al. (2004)	50–74 years of age in population	(I) gFOBT (Hemoccult) (II) FIT (Magstream)	ICER *10 years of biennial screening* (II)/(I): EU 7458/LYS *20 years of biennial screening* (II)/(I): EU 2980/LYS
UK Whynes and Nottingham (2004)	45–74 years of age in asymptomatic population	(I) Biennial FOBT (II) No screen	ICER (I)/(II): EU 1584/LYS
US Maciosek et al. (2006)	50 years and older of age in the general population	(I) Screening strategies (annual FOBT; FS every 5 years; colonoscopy every 10 years) (II) no screen	ICER (I)/(II): 11,900/LYS (weighted average of these three strategies)
US Lairson et al. (2008)	50–74 years of age	(I) Standard intervention (SI) group: Mailed standard intervention; stool blood testing (SBT) screening and FS screening examination (II) tailored intervention (TI) group: Standard intervention plus 2 tailored "message pages."(III) tailored intervention plus a telephone call (TIP) group) (IV) usual care	ICER (I)/(IV): 319/LYS (II)/(I): Dominated (III)/(I): 5843/LYS

Country/Author/ Year	Target population	Strategies	Outcome measures/results
US Lansdorp-Vogelaar et al. (2009a)	50–80 years of age in general population	(I) Optical colonoscopy (II) CTC with referral to optical colonoscopy of any suspected polyp (III) CTC with referral to optical colonoscopy of a suspected polyp ≥6 mm (IV) CTC with referral to optical colonoscopy of a suspected polyp ≥10 mm.	ICER (II-IV)/(I): ICER < $373/LYS
US Lansdorp-Vogelaar et al. (2009b)	50–80 years of age in general population	(I) Annual gFOBT (II) annual FIT (III) FS every 5 years (IV) (III) + (I) (V) colonoscopy every 10 years	Compared with no screening, the treatment savings from preventing advanced colorectal cancer and colorectal cancer deaths (average savings vs costs per individual in the population), (I): $1398 vs $859/per individual (II): $1756 vs $1565/per individual (III): $1706 vs $1575/per individual (IV): $1931 vs $1878/per individual (V): Not cost saving
US Lansdorp-Vogelaar et al. (2010)	65 years of age (Medicare eligible) individuals	(I) Stool DNA test every 3 years (II) stool DNA test every 5 years (III) currently-recommended screening strategies (IV) no screen	ICER(I)/(IV): $14,105/LYS(II)/ (IV): $11,375/LYScompared with (III), (I) and (II) are dominated.
Canada Telford et al. (2010)	50 years of age in the general population	(I) Annual gFOBT (II) annual FIT (III) colonoscopy every 10 years (IV) no screen	ICER (I)/(IV): CAD 9159/QALY (II)/(I):CAD 611/QALY (III)/(II): CAD 6133/QALY
France Berchi et al. (2010)	50–74 years of age in the general population	(I) One round screening: gFOBT (II) one round screening: FIT	ICER (I)/(II): EUD −47,555 ~ 7223/ advanced tumor screened
France Lejeune et al. (2010)	50–74 years of age in the general population	(I) Biennial three-stool unrehydrated gFOBT (Hemoccult-II) (II) biennial FIT (instant-view) (III) no screen	ICER (I)/(III): EUD 2739/LYS (II)/(III): EUD 2819/LYS (II)/(I): EUD 2988/LYS
US Knudsen et al. (2010)	65 years of age and older in average-risk Medicare population.	(I) CTC every 5 years (II) no screen	ICER (I)/(II): ICER<$10,000/LYS, range from $1800 to $9500/LYS
Netherlands Lansdorp-Vogelaar et al. (2011)	Systematic reviews of cost-effectiveness studies between 1993 and 2009 in average-risk populations.	(I) gFOBT (II) FIT (III) FS every 5 years (IV) Colonoscopy every 10 years (V) Stool DNA test (VI) CTC (VII) No screen	ICER(II)/(I): $3900/LYS or dominant (dominated by SENSA) (II)/(I, III, IV, V, VI, VII): Dominant (V)/(I, II, III, IV, VI, VII): Dominated (VI)/(III): Dominant (VI)/(IV): $14,600–$74,200/LYS or dominated (VI)/(I) + (III): Dominated
Netherland Wilschut et al. (2011)	45–80 years of age in the general population	FIT with different starting age, inter-screening interval	ICER For each strategy, compared with next cheaper strategy: ICER < EU $20,000/LYS

Country/Author/Year	Target population	Strategies	Outcome measures/results
Netherlands van Rossum et al. (2011)	50–75 years of age in the general population	(I) One round screening: FIT (II) one round screening: gFOBT (III) No screen	ICER (I)/(II): Dominant (I)/(III): Dominant
Iceland Sharp et al. (2012)	55–74 years of age in the general population	(I) Biennial FIT (II) Annual gFOBT (III) Oneshot FS at 60 years of age(IV) No screen	ICER (III)/(IV): EUD 589/QALY (I)/(IV): EUD 1696/QALY (II)/(IV): EUD 4428/QALY
Israel Ginsberg et al. (2012)	50 years of age and older in developing countries (sub-Saharan Africa and South East Asia)	(I) Annual FOBT (II) FS every 5 years (III) Colonoscopy every 10 years (IV) No screen	ICER *Sub-Saharan Africa:* (III)/(IV): $9598/QALY (I) + (II)/(IV): $15,548/QALY *South East Asia:* (III)/(IV): $28,017/QALY (I) + (II)/(IV): $42,940/QALY
Italy Hassan et al. (2012)	50–80 years of age in the general population	(I) Colonoscopy by nongastroenterologists (II) Colonoscopy by gastroenterologists (III) No screen	ICER (I) + (II)/(III): 5091/LYS (I)/(III): 6332/LYS (II)/(III): 4351/LYS
Singapore Dan et al. (2012)	50–75 years of age in the general population	(I) Oneshot FS at 60 years of age (II) Oneshot colonoscopy at 60 years of age (III) Annual FIT (IV) DCBE every 5 years (V) FS every 5 years (VI) CTC every 5 years(VII) Colonoscopy every 10 years(VIII) Stool DNA test every 5 years (IX) No screen	ICER (I)/(IX): USD$27,843/QALY (III)/(IX): USD$27,399/QALY (IV)/(IX): USD$38,385/QALY (II)/(IX): USD$37,516/QALY (V)/(IX): USD$38,280/ QALY(V) + (III)/(IX): USD$40,000/QALY(VIII)/(IX): USD$46,900/QALY(VII)/(IX): USD$33,720/QALY(VI)/(IX): USD$49,580/QALY
US Hassan et al. (2012)	50–80 years of age in the general population	(I) Aspirin chemoprophylaxis (II) FS (III) Colonoscopy (IV) No screen	ICER (I)/(IV): Dominant (II)/(IV): USD 7434/LYS (I) + (II)/(IV): USD 6511/LYS (III)/(IV): USD 6307/LYS (I) + (III)/(IV): USD 6237/LYS
Ireland Hanly et al. (2012)	Systematic review of cost-effectiveness or cost-utility analyses of CT-colonography-based screening, published in English, January 1999–July 2010.	I. CTC II. FS III. FOBT IV. FIT V. colonoscopy VI. No screening	Incremental cost-effectiveness ratio (V)/(I): US$10,408–$63,900/LYS, (I)/(V): US$23,234/LYS (5 year), US$2144/LYS (10 year) (I)/(II): Dominant (I)/(VI): US $17,672/LYS(I)/(II) + (III): Dominant
US Dinh et al. (2012)	50 years of age in the general population	I. Colonoscopy II. No screening	ICER With history of diabetes at baseline (I)/(II): US$ 6209–270,005/QALY (when the screening stop age is increased, ICER is increased) Without history of diabetes at baseline (I)/(II): US$ 5937–77,500/QALY (when the screening stop age is increased, ICER is increased)

Country/Author/Year	Target population	Strategies	Outcome measures/results
US Behl et al. (2012)	Patients with metastatic colorectal cancer	I. Screening for KRAS and BRAF mutations testing II. Screening for KRAS mutations testing III. Anti-EGFR therapy IV. No anti-EGFR therapy	Incremental cost-effectiveness ratio (I) + (III)/(IV): USD$648,396/LYS (II) + (III)/(IV): USD$2,814,338/LYS (III)/(IV): USD$2,932,767/LYS
US Sharaf and Ladabaum (2013)	50 years of age in the general population	I. Annual FOBT II. Annual FIT III. FS every 5 years IV. FS every 5 years and FIT every 3 years V. Colonoscopy every 10 yearsVI. FS once at aged 60VII. No screening	ICER (V)/(VII): US$2640/QALY(I).(II).(III).(IV).(VI)/(VII): Dominant (III)/(VI): US$1700/QALY (V)/(VI): US$9600/QALY (IV)/(VI): US$2580/QALY (I)/(VI): Dominant (III)/(I): US$105000/QALY (V)/(I): US$67300/QALY (IV)/(I): US$23200/QALY V)/(III): US$56800/QALY (IV)/(III): US$6660/QALY (II)/(I).(IV).(V).(VI): Dominant (IV)/(V):Dominant (IV)/(II): US$271000/QALY
Germany Ladabaum et al. (2013)	50–80 years of age in the general population	I. (Methylated Septin 9 DNA; SEPT9II. Annual FOBT III. Annual FIT IV. FS every 5 years V. Colonoscopy every 10 years VI. No screening	ICER (I)/(II), (III), (IV), (V): Dominant (III)/(I),(II), (IV), (V), (VI): Dominated (I)/(VI): US$8400–11,500/QALY
US Pence et al. (2013)	50–75 years of age in the general population	I. ColonoscopyII. Colonoscopy + aspirinIII. Colonoscopy + calcium IV. Colonoscopy + aspirin + calciumIV. No screening	ICER (I)/(V): Dominant (II)/(I): US$12,950/LYS, $3061/CFYS(cancer-free years saved) (III)/(I): US$13,041/LYS, $2317/CFYS (IV)/(I): US$26,269/LYS, $6244/CFYS
US Dinh et al. (2013)	50–75 years of age in the general population	I. Colonoscopy II. FIT III. Sigmoidoscopy IV. II + III V. Annual FIT + colonoscopy (aged 66) VI. No screening	ICER (I),(II),(III),(IV),(V)/(VI): Dominant (I),(II),(IV),(V)/(III): Dominant (V)/(II): US$9700/QALY (IV)/(II): US$9900/QALY (I)/(II): US$16400/QALY (IV)/(V): US$11300/QALY (I)/(V): US$35100/QALY (I)/(IV): US$51000/QALY
Netherlands Goede et al. (2013)	55–75 years of age in the general population	I. One-sample FIT II. Two-sample FIT III. No screening	ICER (I)/(III): EUD 2690–3473/LYS (II)/(I): EUD 16818–31,930/LYS (Two positive sample); EUD 4024–8041/LYS (at least one positive sample)

Country/Author/Year	Target population	Strategies	Outcome measures/results
Netherlands Van Hees et al. (2014)	Unscreened elderly aged 76–90	I. Once-only colonoscopy screening II. Once-only sigmoidoscopy screening III. Once-only FIT screening IV. No screening	ICER *No comorbidity* (II)/(IV): $8000–$208,000/QALY (aged 76–86) (I)/(IV): $21,000–$261,000/QALY (aged 76–86) (III)/(IV): $15,000–$86,000/QALY (aged 76–86; aged 76–78 dominated) *Moderate comorbidity* (II)/(IV): $23,000–$174,000/QALY (aged 76–86) (I)/(IV): $45,000–$230,000/QALY (aged 76–86) (III)/(IV): $21,000–$83,000/QALY (aged 76–86) *Severe comorbidity* (II)/(IV): $50,000–$139,000/QALY (aged 76–86) (I)/(IV): $83,000–$185,000/QALY (aged 76–86) (III)/(IV): $39,000–$78,000/QALY (aged 76–86)
US Ladabaum et al. (2014)	50–75 years of age in the general population	I. FOBT: Aged 50–54 every year, aged 55-7 every 2 years II. FOBT/COLO 55.65: Aged 50–54 FOBT every year, aged 55.65 colonoscopy III. FOBT/COLO 60.70: Aged 50–54 FOBT every year, aged 60.70 colonoscopy IV. FIT: Aged 50–54 FIT every year, aged 55–75 FIT every 2 years V. FIT/COLO 55.65: Aged 50–54 FIT every year, aged 55.65 colonoscopy VI. FIT/COLO 60.70: Aged 50–54 FIT every year, aged 60.70 colonoscopy VII. COLO 55.65: Aged 55.65 colonoscopy VIII. COLO 60.70: Aged 60.70 colonoscopy IX. Methylated Septin 9 DNA (every year or every 2 years) X. No screening	ICER (IX)/(X): EU$600–3600/QALY (I–VIII)/(X): Dominant (IX)/(VIII): EU$42700–1,600,000/QALY (I)/(VIII): EU$14900/QALY (II-VII)/(VIII) dominant (I-VIII)/(IX) dominant(IX)/(I): EU$49400–124,300/QALY (II-VII)/(I) dominant (IX)/(VII): EU$149000–890,000/QALY (II-VI)/(VII) dominant (IX)/(III): EU$173000–1,600,000/QALY (II)/(III): EU$1200/QALY (V)/(III): EU$2400/QALY (VI).(IV)/(III) dominate (II)/(VI): EU$85700/QALY (V)/(VI): EU$9500/QALY (IV)/(VI): dominate (IV)/(II): dominate (V)/(II): EU$10300/QALY (V)/(IV): US$12200/QALY

Country/Author/Year	Target population	Strategies	Outcome measures/results
France Lejeune et al. (2014)	50–74 years of age in the general population	I. Unrehydrated gFOBT II. FIT (Magstream, FOB-gold and OC-sensor)	ICER (II: FOB-gold)/(I): Dominate (one stool-sample FOB-gold at 176 ng/ml) (II: FOB-gold)/(I): EU$1108–1687/LYS (two stool-sample FOB-gold at 352–176 ng/ml. When the cut-off is decreased, the ICER is increased.) (II: Magstream)/(I): Dominate (one-stool sample Magstream at 20 ng/ml) (II: Magstream)/(I): EU$1151/LYS (two-stool sample Magstream at 20 ng/ml) (II: OC-sensor)/(I): EU$1595/LYS (one-stool sample OC-sensor at 150 ng/ml) (II: OC-sensor)/(I): EU$3115–3270/LYS (two-stool sample OC-sensor at 300–150 ng/ml. When the cut-off is decreased, the ICER is increased.)
Hong Kong Wong et al. (2015)	50–75 years of age in the general population	I. Annual g-FOBT II. Biennial g-FOBT III. Annual FIT. IV. Biennial FIT V. Colonoscopy every 10 years VI. No screening	ICER (II)/(VI): $5240/QALY(I)/(VI): $5871/QALY (V)/(VI): $3622/QALY (IV)/(VI): $2976/QALY (III)/(VI): $3155/QALY (I)/(II): $7096/QALY (V)/(II): $1831/QALY (IV)/(II): $911/QALY (III)/(II): $1763/QALY (III–IV)/(I) dominate (IV)/(V): dominate (III)/(V): $1659/QALY (III)/(IV): $4087/QALY
UK Patel and Kilgore (2015)	Systematic review for cost-effectiveness analyses focused on CRC screening strategies in the United States and published between May 2007 and February 2014.	I. Annual FOBT II. Annual FOBT III. FS every 5 or 10 years IV. Combination FS every 5 years and annual FOBT or annual FIT V. colonoscopy every 10 years VI. Virtual colonoscopy every 5 or 10 years VII. Stool DNA test every 2, 3, or 5 years VIII. No screening	ICER (VII)/(VIII): $34,258/LYS (I–VI)/(VIII): ICER<$20,000/LYS (IV)/(VIII): ICER<$15,000/LYS or dominant (III)/(VIII): ICER<$10,000/LYS (FS every 10 years) (V)/(VIII): ICER<$28,000/LYS dominant (beginning at 50 years of age) (VI)/(VIII): ICER<$22,000/LYS (virtual colonoscopy every 5 years); ICER<$23,000/LYS (virtual colonoscopy every 10 years, dominant in 1 study) (VII)/(VIII): ICER<$35,000/LYS
US van Hees et al. (2015)	Unscreened elderly aged 76–90	I. Once only colonoscopy II. No screening	Incremental cost-effectiveness ratio (I): $22,000/QALY (women aged 66 years) ~ $4,000,000/QALY (women aged 84 years)

Country/Author/ Year	Target population	Strategies	Outcome measures/results
UK Asaria et al. (2015)	60–74 years of age in the general population	I. Biennial gFOBT II. (I) + target reminder III. (I) + universal reminder (universal basic reminder letter all eligible patients). IV. No screening	Incremental net health benefit (λ = EU$20000/QALY) (I)/(IV): 40372 QALY (II)/(IV): 41581 QALY (III)/(IV): 42642 QALY
Hong Kong Lam et al. (2015)	50–75 years of age in the general population	I. Annual g-FOBT II. Annual FIT, III. Biennial G-FOBT, IV. Biennial I-FOBT, V. FS every 5 years, VI. FS every 10 years, VII. Colonoscopy every 5 year VIII. Colonoscopy every 10 years, IX. No screening	ICER (I)/(IX): HK$151000/QALY (II)/(IX): HK$52000/QALY (III)/(IX): HK$129000/QALY (IV)/(IX): HK$44000/QALY (V)/(IX): HK$144000/QALY (VI)/(IX): HK$139000/QALY (VII)/(IX): HK$131000/QALY (VIII)/(IX): HK$116000/QALY (I) + (V)/(IX): HK$186000/QALY (I) + (VI)/(IX): HK$179000/QALY (II) + (V)/(IX): HK$105000/QALY (II) + (VI)/(IX): HK$81000/QALY
Hong Kong Wong et al. (2016)	50–70 years of age in the general population	I. FS 5 yearly II. Colonoscopy 10 yearly III. FS for each woman at 50- and 55-year old followed by colonoscopy at 60- and 70-year old; male subjects received colonoscopy at 50-, 60-, and 70-year old; IV. FS for each woman at 50-, 55-, 60, and 65-year old followed by colonoscopy at 70-year old; male subjects received colonoscopy at 50-, 60-, and 70-year old; V. FS for each woman at 50-, 55-, 60-, 65-, and 70-year old; male subjects received colonoscopy at 50-, 60-, and 70-year old. VI. No screening	ICER (I)/(VI): US$56510/LYS (II)/(VI): US$43739/LYS (III)/(VI): US$43517/LYS (IV)/(VI): US$47710/LYS (V)/(VI): US$42515/LYS
Belgium Pil et al. (2016)	50 years of age in the general population	I. FIT II. No screening	ICER (I)/(II): EU$1681/QALY (male); EU$4484/QALY (female)
US Ladabaum and Mannalithara (2016)	50–80 years of age in the general population	I. Multitarget stool DNA (MT-sDNA) every 3 years II. FIT every 2 years or yearly III. Colonoscopy every 10 years IV. No screening	ICER (II)/(IV): Dominant (I)/(IV): $29,500/QALY (III)/(IV): $15,000/QALY (I)/(II)-2 yr.: $2,390,000/QALY (III)/(II)-2 yr.: $43,600/QALY (II)-1 yr./(II)-2 yr.: $33,000/QALY (III)/(I) dominant (II)-1 yr./(I) dominant (II)-1 yr./(III): Dominant
Japan Sekiguchi et al. (2016)	Average-risk population aged 40 years or over.	I.FIT II. Colonoscopy III. Aged 40–49 years: FIT, Aged 50 years: Colonoscopy IV. No screening	ICER (I-III)/(IV) dominant (II)/(I): JP $293,616/QALY (III)/(I): Dominant (II)/(III): JP $781,342/QALY

Country/Author/Year	Target population	Strategies	Outcome measures/results
Netherlands Greuter et al. (2017)	Asymptomatic persons aged 55–75 years without a prior CRC diagnosis	I. FIT without colonoscopy surveillance II. FIT with colonoscopy surveillance III. No screening	ICER (III)/(I): Dominated (II)/(I): ICER>EU$36602/LYS
UK Murphy et al. (2017)	60–74 years of age in the general population	I. FIT II. gFOBT	ICER (I)/(II): Dominant (for all positive cut-off of FIT) Incremental net benefit compared with gFOBT EU $315–1378/QALY (the lower positive cut-off of FIT, the larger INB)
Sweden Aronsson et al. (2017)	60 years of age in the general population	I. FIT twice II. Repeated FIT (biennial) III. Colonoscopy once IV. Repeated colonoscopy (10 years) V. no screening	ICER (I)/(V): –$700/QALY (III)/(V): –$1300/QALY (II)/(V): $2700/QALY (IV)/(V): $2200/QALY (III)/(I): Dominated (II)/(III): $81,500/QALY (IV)/(III): $26,900/QALY (II)/(I): $6200/QALY (IV)/(I): $4800/QALY
Netherlands Naber et al. (2018)	50 years of age in the general population with affected first-degree relatives	I. Colonoscopy every 10 years starting at age 50 for people with at least one affected first-degree relatives II. No screening	ICER (I)/(II): $1000–185,000/QALY (the larger number of affected FDRs at age 50, the lower ICER. If the number of affected FDRs equal or larger than 4, this strategy is potentially cost-saving.
Netherlands Lansdorp-Vogelaar et al. (2018)	General population	I. Fecal immunochemical test; II. Biomarker test	ICER (II)/(I): ICER>EU$50000/LYS
US Subramanian et al. (2017)	50 years of age in the general population and individuals with strong family history (two or more relatives with colorectal cancer, or one relative diagnosed before the age of 50)	I. Present strategy: Majority of individuals are considered average risk and begin screening at age 50 using either colonoscopy or fecal tests. II. Personalized strategy: Individuals are assigned to the five risk categories and screening schedule is based on assigned risk category[a] III. Future strategy (II+ biomarker testing).	Incremental cost per life years gained (II)/(I): $18342–23,961/LYS (from 60 to 80% compliance rates. When compliance is increased to 80%, ICER is increased; if the compliance rate is 100%, it is dominated.) (III)/(I): $47108–199,366/LYS from 60 to 100% compliance rates. When compliance is increased to 100%, ICER is increased)

Increased: Colonoscopy every 5 years starting at age 40

Medium: Colonoscopy every 10 years or fecal test annually starting at age 50

Decreased: Colonoscopy at age 50 only, or fecal test every 2 years starting at age 50

Low: 30% Colonoscopy at age 50 only

CTC Computed tomographic colonography, *DCBE* Double-contrast barium enema, *FIT* fecal immunochemical test, *FOBT* faecal occult blood test, *FS* Flexible sigmoidoscopy, *gFOBT* Guaiac-based FOBT

[a]High: Colonoscopy every 2 years starting at age 20

References

Allison JE, Tekawa IS, Ransom LJ, Adrain AL. A comparison of fecal occult-blood tests for colorectal-cancer screening. N Engl J Med. 1996;334(3):155–9.

Aronsson M, Carlsson P, Levin LÅ, Hager J, Hultcrantz R. Cost-effectiveness of high-sensitivity faecal immunochemical test and colonoscopy screening for colorectal cancer. Br J Surg. 2017;104(8):1078–86.

Asaria M, Griffin S, Cookson R, Whyte S, Tappenden P. Distributional cost-effectiveness analysis of health care programmes--a methodological case study of the UK bowel Cancer screening Programme. Health Econ. 2015;24(6):742–54.

Behl AS, Goddard KA, Flottemesch TJ, Veenstra D, Meenan RT, Lin JS, Maciosek MV. Cost-effectiveness analysis of screening for KRAS and BRAF mutations in metastatic colorectal cancer. J Natl Cancer Inst. 2012;104(23):1785–95.

Benson VS, Patnick J, Davies AK, Nadel MR, Smith RA, Atkin WS. CRC screening: a comparison of 35 initiatives in 17 countries. Int J Cancer. 2008;122(6):1357–67.

Berchi C, Bouvier V, Réaud JM, Launoy G. Cost-effectiveness analysis of two strategies for mass screening for colorectal cancer in France. Health Econ. 2004;13(3):227–38.

Berchi C, Guittet L, Bouvier V, Launoy G. Cost-effectiveness analysis of the optimal threshold of an automated immunochemical test for colorectal cancer screening: performances of immunochemical colorectal cancer screening. Int J Technol Assess Health Care. 2010;26(1):48–53.

Briggs AH, O'Brien BJ, Blackhouse G. Thinking outside the box: recent advances in the analysis and presentation of uncertainty in cost-effectiveness studies. Annu Rev Public Health. 2002;23:377–401.

Chen THH, Chiu YH, Luh DL, Yen MF, Wu HM, Chen LS, Tung TH, et al. Community-based multiple screening model: design, implementation, and analysis of 42387 participants Taiwan community-based integrated screening group. Cancer. 2004;100(8):1734–43.

Chen LS, Liao CS, Chang SH, Lai HC, Chen THH. Cost-effectiveness analysis for determining optimal cut-off of immunochemical faecal occult blood test for population-based CRC screening (KCIS 16). J Med Screen. 2007;14(4):191–9.

Cheng TI, Wong JM, Hong CF, et al. Colorectal cancer screening in asymptomaic adults: comparison of colonoscopy, sigmoidoscopy and fecal occult blood tests. J Formos Med Assoc. 2002;101:685–90.

Dan YY, Chuah BY, Koh DC, Yeoh KG. Screening based on risk for colorectal cancer is the most cost-effective approach. Clin Gastroenterol Hepatol. 2012;10(3):266–71.e1–6.

Dinh TA, Alperin P, Walter LC, Smith R. Impact of comorbidity on colorectal cancer screening cost-effectiveness study in diabetic populations. J Gen Intern Med. 2012;27(6):730–8.

Dinh T, Ladabaum U, Alperin P, Caldwell C, Smith R, Levin TR. Health benefits and cost-effectiveness of a hybrid screening strategy for colorectal cancer. Clin Gastroenterol Hepatol. 2013;11(9):1158–66.

Frazier AL, Colditz GA, Fuchs CS, Kuntz KM. Cost-effectiveness of screening for colorectal cancer in the general population. JAMA. 2000;284(15):1954–61.

Ginsberg GM, Lauer JA, Zelle S, Baeten S, Baltussen R. Cost effectiveness of strategies to combat breast, cervical, and colorectal cancer in sub-Saharan Africa and South East Asia: mathematical modelling study. BMJ. 2012;344:e614.

Goede SL, van Roon AH, Reijerink JC, van Vuuren AJ, Lansdorp-Vogelaar I, Habbema JD, Kuipers EJ, van Leerdam ME, van Ballegooijen M. Cost-effectiveness of one versus two sample faecal immunochemical testing for colorectal cancer screening. Gut. 2013;62(5):727–34.

Green PD, Bertario L, Gnauck R, Kronborg O, Hardcastle JD, Epstein MS, Sadowski D, Sudduth R, Zuckerman GR, Rockey DC. A prospective multicenter evaluation of new fecal occult blood tests in patients undergoing colonoscopy. Am J Gastroenterol. 2000;95(5):1331–8.

Greuter MJE, de Klerk CM, Meijer GA, Dekker E, Coupé VMH. Screening for colorectal Cancer with fecal immunochemical testing with and without Postpolypectomy surveillance colonoscopy: a cost-effectiveness analysis. Ann Intern Med. 2017;167(8):544–54.

Hanly P, Skally M, Fenlon H, Sharp L. Cost-effectiveness of computed tomography colonography in colorectal cancer screening: a systematic review. Int J Technol Assess Health Care. 2012;28(4):415–23.

Hardcastle JD, Chamberlain JO, Robinson MH, Moss SM, Amar SS, Balfour TW, James PD, Mangham CM. Randomised controlled trial of faecal-occult-blood screening for colorectal cancer. The Lancet. 1996;348(9040):1472–7.

Hassan C, Rex DK, Zullo A, Cooper GS. Loss of efficacy and cost-effectiveness when screening colonoscopy is performed by nongastroenterologists. Cancer. 2012;118(18):4404–11.

Knudsen AB, Lansdorp-Vogelaar I, Rutter CM, Savarino JE, van Ballegooijen M, Kuntz KM, Zauber AG. Cost-effectiveness of computed tomographic colonography screening for colorectal cancer in the Medicare population. J Natl Cancer Inst. 2010 Aug 18;102(16):1238–52.

Kronborg O, Fenger C, Olsen J, Jørgensen OD, Søndergaard O. Randomised study of screening for colorectal cancer with faecal-occult-blood test. The Lancet. 1996;348(9040):1467–71.

Ladabaum U, Mannalithara A. Comparative effectiveness and cost effectiveness of a multitarget stool DNA test to screen for colorectal neoplasia. Gastroenterology. 2016;151(3):427–39.

Ladabaum U, Chopra CL, Huang G, Scheiman JM, Chernew ME, Fendrick AM. Aspirin as an adjunct to screening for prevention of sporadic colorectal cancer. A cost-effectiveness analysis. Ann Intern Med. 2001;135(9):769–81.

Ladabaum U, Allen J, Wandell M, Ramsey S. Colorectal cancer screening with blood-based biomarkers: cost-effectiveness of methylated septin 9 DNA versus current strategies. Cancer Epidemiol Biomark Prev. 2013;22(9):1567–76.

Ladabaum U, Alvarez-Osorio L, Rösch T, Brueggenjuergen B. Cost-effectiveness of colorectal cancer screening in Germany: current endoscopic and fecal testing strategies versus plasma methylated Septin 9 DNA. Endosc Int Open. 2014;2(2):E96–E104.

Lairson DR, DiCarlo M, Myers RE, Wolf T, Cocroft J, Sifri R, Rosenthal M, Vernon SW, Wender R. Cost-effectiveness of targeted and tailored interventions on colorectal cancer screening use. Cancer. 2008;112(4):779–88.

Lam CL, Law WL, Poon JT, Chan P, Wong CK, McGhee SM, Fong DY. Health-related quality of life in patients with colorectal neoplasm and cost-effectiveness of colorectal cancer screening in Hong Kong. Hong Kong Med J. 2015;21(Suppl 6):4–8.

Lansdorp-Vogelaar I, van Ballegooijen M, Zauber AG, Boer R, Wilschut J, Habbema JD. At what costs will screening with CT colonography be competitive? A cost-effectiveness approach. Int J Cancer. 2009a;124(5):1161–8.

Lansdorp-Vogelaar I, van Ballegooijen M, Zauber AG, Habbema JD, Kuipers EJ. Effect of rising chemotherapy costs on the cost savings of colorectal cancer screening. J Natl Cancer Inst. 2009b;101(20):1412–22.

Lansdorp-Vogelaar I, Kuntz KM, Knudsen AB, Wilschut JA, Zauber AG, van Ballegooijen M. Stool DNA testing to screen for colorectal cancer in the Medicare population: a cost-effectiveness analysis. Ann Intern Med. 2010;153(6):368–77.

Lansdorp-Vogelaar I, Knudsen AB, Brenner H. Cost-effectiveness of colorectal cancer screening. Epidemiol Rev. 2011;33:88–100.

Lansdorp-Vogelaar I, Goede SL, Bosch LJW, Melotte V, Carvalho B, van Engeland M, Meijer GA, de Koning HJ, van Ballegooijen M. Cost-effectiveness of high-performance biomarker tests vs fecal immunochemical test for noninvasive colorectal Cancer screening. Clin Gastroenterol Hepatol. 2018;16(4):504–12.

Lejeune C, Dancourt V, Arveux P, Bonithon-Kopp C, Faivre J. Cost-effectiveness of screening for colorectal cancer in France using a guaiac test versus an immunochemical test. Int J Technol Assess Health Care. 2010;26(1):40–7.

Lejeune C, Le Gleut K, Cottet V, Galimard C, Durand G, Dancourt V, Faivre J. The cost-effectiveness of immunochemical tests for colorectal cancer screening. Dig Liver Dis. 2014;46(1):76–81.

Levi Z, Rozen P, Hazazi R, et al. A quantitative immunochemical fecal occult blood test for colorectal neoplasia. Ann Intern Med. 2007;146:244–55.

Maciosek MV, Solberg LI, Coffield AB, Edwards NM, Goodman MJ. Colorectal cancer screening: health impact and cost effectiveness. Am J Prev Med. 2006;31(1):80–9.

Mandel JS, Bond JH, Church TR, Snover DC, Bradley GM, Schuman LM, Ederer F. Reducing mortality from colorectal cancer by screening for fecal occult blood. N Engl J Med. 1993;328(19):1365–71.

McMahon PM, Bosch JL, Gleason S, Halpern EF, Lester JS, Gazelle GS. Cost-effectiveness of colorectal cancer screening. Radiology. 2001;219(1):44–50.

Murphy J, Halloran S, Gray A. Cost-effectiveness of the faecal immunochemical test at a range of positivity thresholds compared with the guaiac faecal occult blood test in the NHS bowel Cancer screening Programme in England. BMJ Open. 2017;7(10):e017186.

Naber SK, Kuntz KM, Henrikson NB, Williams MS, Calonge N, Goddard KAB, Zallen DT, Ganiats TG, Webber EM, Janssens ACJW, van Ballegooijen M, Zauber AG, Lansdorp-Vogelaar I. Cost effectiveness of age-specific screening intervals for people with family histories of colorectal Cancer. Gastroenterology. 2018;154(1):105–16.

Patel SS, Kilgore ML. Cost effectiveness of colorectal Cancer screening strategies. Cancer Control. 2015;22(2):248–58.

Pence BC, Belasco EJ, Lyford CP. Combination aspirin and/or calcium chemoprevention with colonoscopy in colorectal cancer prevention: cost-effectiveness analyses. Cancer Epidemiol Biomark Prev. 2013;22(3):399–405.

Pil L, Fobelets M, Putman K, Trybou J, Annemans L. Cost-effectiveness and budget impact analysis of a population-based screening program for colorectal cancer. Eur J Intern Med. 2016;32:72–8.

Salkeld G, Young G, Irwig L, Haas M, Glasziou P. Cost-effectiveness analysis of screening by faecal occult blood testing for colorectal cancer in Australia. Aust N Z J Public Health. 1996;20(2):138–43.

Sekiguchi M, Igarashi A, Matsuda T, Matsumoto M, Sakamoto T, Nakajima T, Kakugawa Y, Yamamoto S, Saito H, Saito Y. Optimal use of colonoscopy and fecal immunochemical test for population-based colorectal cancer screening: a cost-effectiveness analysis using Japanese data. Jpn J Clin Oncol. 2016;46(2):116–25.

Sharaf RN, Ladabaum U. Comparative effectiveness and cost-effectiveness of screening colonoscopy vs. sigmoidoscopy and alternative strategies. Am J Gastroenterol. 2013;108(1):120–32.

Sharp L, Tilson L, Whyte S, O'Ceilleachair A, Walsh C, Usher C, Tappenden P, Chilcott J, Staines A, Barry M, Comber H. Cost-effectiveness of population-based screening for colorectal cancer: a comparison of guaiac-based faecal occult blood testing, faecal immunochemical testing and flexible sigmoidoscopy. Br J Cancer. 2012;106(5):805–16.

Sonnenberg A, Delcò F, Inadomi JM. Cost-effectiveness of colonoscopy in screening for colorectal cancer. Ann Intern Med. 2000;133(8):573–84.

Subramanian S, Bobashev G, Morris RJ, Hoover S. Personalized medicine for prevention: can risk stratified screening decrease colorectal cancer mortality at an acceptable cost? Cancer Causes Control. 2017;28(4):299–308.

Suleiman S, Rex DK, Sonnenberg A. Chemoprevention of colorectal cancer by aspirin: a cost-effectiveness analysis. Gastroenterology. 2002;122(1):78–84.

Telford JJ, Levy AR, Sambrook JC, Zou D, Enns RA. The cost-effectiveness of screening for colorectal cancer. CMAJ. 2010;182(12):1307–13.

van Ballegooijen M, Habbema JDF, Boer R, Zauber AG, Brown ML. Report to the Agency for Healthcare Research and Quality: a comparison of the cost-effectiveness of fecal occult blood tests with different test characteristics in the context of annual screening in the Medicare population. Agency for Healthcare Research and Quality, 2003.

van Hees F, Habbema JD, Meester RG, Lansdorp-Vogelaar I, van Ballegooijen M, Zauber AG. Should colorectal cancer screening be considered in elderly persons without previous screening? A cost-effectiveness analysis. Ann Intern Med. 2014;160(11):750–9.

van Hees F, Saini SD, Lansdorp-Vogelaar I, Vijan S, Meester RG, de Koning HJ, Zauber AG, van Ballegooijen M. Personalizing colonoscopy screening for elderly individuals based on screening history, cancer risk, and comorbidity status could increase cost effectiveness. Gastroenterology. 2015;149(6):1425–37.

van Rossum LG, van Rijn AF, Verbeek AL, van Oijen MG, Laheij RJ, Fockens P, Jansen JB, Adang EM, Dekker E. Colorectal cancer screening comparing no screening, immunochemical and guaiac fecal occult blood tests: a cost-effectiveness analysis. Int J Cancer. 2011 Apr 15;128(8):1908–17.

Weinstein MC, Finberg HV. Clinical decision analysis. Philadelphia: Saunders; 1980.

Whitlock EP, Lin JS, Liles E, et al. Screening for colorectal cancer: a targeted, updated systematic review for the U.S. preventive services task force. Ann Intern Med. 2008;149:638–58.

Whynes DK, Nottingham FOB. Screening trial. Cost-effectiveness of screening for colorectal cancer: evidence from the Nottingham faecal occult blood trial. J Med Screen. 2004;11(1):11–5.

Wilschut JA, Hol L, Dekker E, Jansen JB, Van Leerdam ME, Lansdorp-Vogelaar I, Kuipers EJ, Habbema JD, Van Ballegooijen M. Cost-cffectiveness analysis of a quantitative immunochemical test for colorectal cancer screening. Gastroenterology. 2011;141(5):1648–55.

Wong CK, Lam CL, Wan YF, Fong DY. Cost-effectiveness simulation and analysis of colorectal cancer screening in Hong Kong Chinese population: comparison amongst colonoscopy, guaiac and immunologic fecal occult blood testing. BMC Cancer. 2015;15:705.

Wong MC, Ching JY, Chan VC, Lam TY, Luk AK, Wong SH, Ng SC, Ng SS, Wu JC, Chan FK, Sung JJ. Colorectal Cancer screening based on age and gender: a cost-effectiveness analysis. Medicine (Baltimore). 2016;95(10):e2739.

Wu GH, Wang YM, Yen AM, Wong JM, Lai HC, Warwick J, Chen TH. Cost-effectiveness analysis of colorectal cancer screening with stool DNA testing in intermediate-incidence countries. BMC Cancer. 2006 May 24;6:136.

Yang KC, Liao CS, Chiu YH, Yen AM, Chen TH. Colorectal cancer screening with faecal occult blood test within a multiple disease screening programme: an experience from Keelung, Taiwan. J Med Screen. 2006;13(Suppl 1):S8–13.

Young GP, St John DJ, Winawer SJ. Rozen P; WHO (World Health Organization) and OMED (world Organization for Digestive Endoscopy). Choice of fecal occult blood tests for colorectal cancer screening: recommendations based on performance characteristics in population studies: a WHO (World Health Organization) and OMED (world Organization for Digestive Endoscopy) report. Am J Gastroenterol. 2002;97(10):2499–507.

Future of Colorectal Cancer Screening: Screening in the Big Data Era and Personalized Screening Strategy

Wen-Feng Hsu, Chen-Yang Hsu, and Hsiu-Hsi Chen

Abstract

Population-based colorectal cancer (CRC) screening with FIT is well established in Western countries. However, its application to the general population is still faced with inaccuracy of FIT and economic concern given scarce resources. To be more precise and efficient, an alternative is to adopt personalized screening strategy by making use of risk stratification computed by the risk assessment multistate model with the incorporation of multifactorial correlates. In this chapter, we design and frame a multistate and multifactorial natural history model to incorporate fecal hemoglobin (f-Hb) concentration, lifestyle factors, comorbidity, chromosomal instability (CSI), and CpG island methylator phenotype (CIMP) in the evolution of colorectal neoplasm. The computer simulation algorithm was developed to yield multistep scores for calculating multistate probabilities of developing colorectal neoplasia, which provide the basis for risk-based individually tailored screening policy and also its efficacy, utilization, and cost-effectiveness analysis compared with universal screening policy. Through this integrated approach, the individually tailored cancer screening under the concept of translational research has been proposed to solve many problems of current universal mass screening for colorectal cancer. We believe the application of personalized information on f-Hb concentration, genetic markers, and nongenetic factors opens a new avenue to develop a novel personalized population-based screening for CRC.

W.-F. Hsu
Graduate Institute of Epidemiology and Preventive Medicine, College of Public Health, National Taiwan University, Taipei, Taiwan

Department of Medicine, National Taiwan University Cancer Center, Taipei, Taiwan

C.-Y. Hsu
Graduate Institute of Epidemiology and Preventive Medicine, College of Public Health, National Taiwan University, Taipei, Taiwan

Master of Public Health Degree Program, National Taiwan University, Taipei, Taiwan

H.-H. Chen (✉)
Institute of Epidemiology and Preventive Medicine, College of Public Health, National Taiwan University, Taipei, Taiwan
e-mail: chenlin@ntu.edu.tw

Keywords

Personalized colorectal cancer screening
Stool-based test · Bleeding phenotype · Fecal hemoglobin concentration · Quantitative fecal immunochemical test

© Springer Nature Singapore Pte Ltd. 2021
H.-M. Chiu, H.-H. Chen (eds.), *Colorectal Cancer Screening*,
https://doi.org/10.1007/978-981-15-7482-5_11

11.1   Introduction

11.1.1 Personalized Screening Strategy for Colorectal Cancer

Population-based colorectal cancer (CRC) screening is well established in Western countries. However, its application to the underlying general population, particularly Asian countries, is still limited in part due to inaccuracy of fecal immunochemical test (FIT) and in part due to scarce resources. False-negative, leading to interval cancer, (Chiu et al. 2013) and false-positive cases resulting from FIT have been well documented. Moreover, the incidence rate of CRC in Asia as a whole compared with Western countries is still relatively low although there has been an increasing time trend over the past decade especially in socioeconomically developed countries. To reduce the inaccuracy and be more efficient in reducing cost, making allowance for clinical capacity of colonoscopy, and facilitating the optimal surveillance, treatment, and therapy, an alternative is to adopt personalized screening strategy by making use of risk stratification computed by the multistep risk assessment model (Jeon et al. 2018; Cenin et al. 2020) based on state-specific factors as described below.

11.1.2 State-Specific Multistate Natural History of Colorectal Neoplasm

To develop an individually-tailored screening for CRC a mathematical model of multistate and multifactorial model is required to incorporate fecal hemoglobin (f-Hb) concentration, lifestyle factors, comorbidity, chromosomal instability (CSI), microsatellite instability (MSI), and CpG island methylator phenotype (CIMP) with the application of three-state Markov model for the natural history of CRC.

There are several constructs involved with the development of colorectal neoplasia through adenoma–carcinoma pathway. They consist of genetic susceptibility, lifestyle, demographics, and intermediate endpoint such as f-Hb. To develop personalize preventive strategies, factors underlying each construct should be superimposed into the map of multistate natural history of colorectal neoplasia.

As far as genetic factors are concerned, the development of fecal DNA markers for the detection of adenoma and invasive CRC include markers related to tumor suppressor (such as APC, DCC, and TP53) and oncogenes (KRAS) related to the pathway chromosome instability, repair genes such as MSH2 related to MSI, and the epigenetic biomarker panel, so-called the CIMP such as SFRP2, TFPI2 GATA4, NDRG4, OSMR, and vimentin based on the review by Young and Bosch and also CNRIP1, FBN1, INA, MAL, SNCA, and SPG20 proposed by Lind et al. (2012) (Young and Bosch 2011; Bosch et al. 2011; Lind et al. 2011). In a similar vein, other nongenetic factors associated with colorectal neoplasia such as f-Hb as mentioned in Chap. 5 and lifestyle factors described in Chap. 1 can be incorporated into multistate natural history of colorectal neoplasm.

To superimpose theses genetic and nongenetic factors into the map of multistate outcome, it is necessary to compare the distribution of each marker across normal, adenoma, and carcinoma so as to assign the role of each marker played in each transition. Genes related to the pathway chromosome instability play a crucial role in occurrence of adenoma.

11.2   Materials and Methods

11.2.1 Study Procedure

We follow the procedure developed by Yen et al. (2014) for the risk stratification for screen-detectable cancers to develop our mathematical model for personalized colorectal cancer screening with FIT (Yen et al. 2014). The six steps were described below.

1. *Model specification.*

    From the beginning, we used a three-state Markov model (Fig. 11.1a) to depicted the disease natural history for colorectal cancer from normal (State 1), through adenoma (State 2), then to invasive CRC (State 3). The de novo

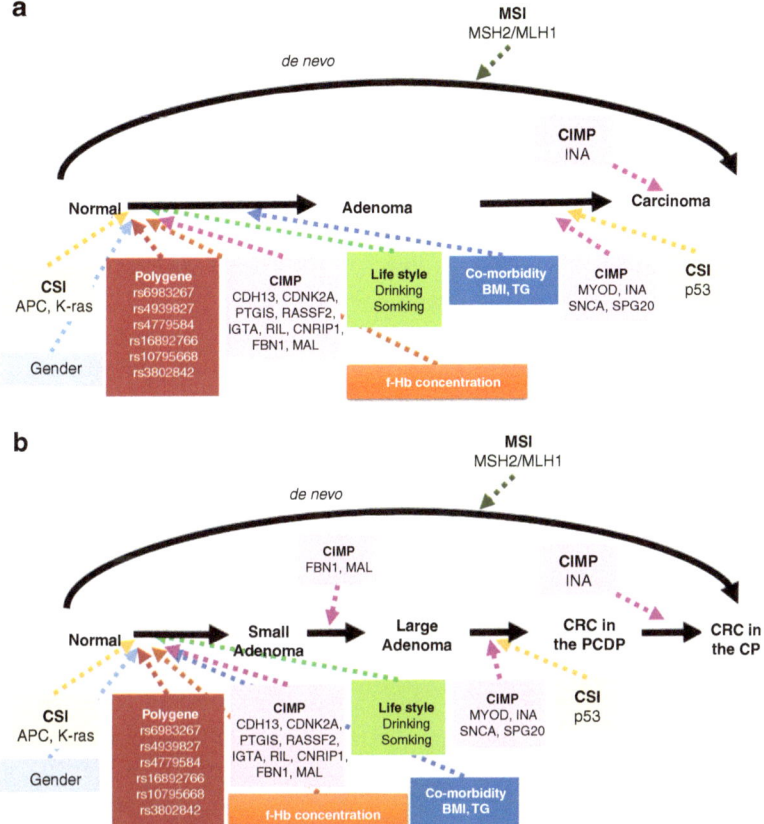

Fig. 11.1 Multistate and multifactorial model for CRC with fecal hemoglobin concentration. (**a**) 3-state Model. (**b**) 5-state Model

pathway for those progressing to malignant exempt of adenoma is also considered. A 5-state Markov model with further classification of adenoma into small and large and CRC into the preclinical detectable phase and the clinical phase (CP) was further considered in order to capture the benefit of CRC screening.

2. *Empirical data.*

We use data from a hospital-based series data for the disease progression for the underlying population (Chen et al. 2003). Because data used were for those first undergoing colonoscopy, we can estimate the natural course of disease progression.

3. *Mapping.*

The possible associated factors were mapped to different transition rates based on

its role in the multistate progression from the literature.

4. *Estimation.*

The transition rates without considering personal characteristics were first estimated with the application of transition probabilities of five-state model following the theory of stochastic process (Cox and Miller 1965). The effects of personal characteristics on different transitions borrowed from the literature were adjusted to tune transition rates estimated from empirical data.

5. *Simulation.*

A hypothetical cohort of 1 million subjects aged 40 years was simulated using a stochastic Monte Carlo simulation. The frequency of f-Hb levels, demographic features, lifestyle, and comorbidity was abstracted from the Taiwanese community. The distribution of polygene, CSI, MSI, and CIMP was from literatures. The risk percentile was determined by the probability of developing colorectal neoplasm. This cohort underwent a study period of 12-year either without screening, or biennial FIT or personalized screening based on his/her risk percentile. We assumed 100% attendance rate. The newly CRC cases during a 12-year follow-up after the study period were collected.

6. *Application.*

The simulation was used to evaluate the effectiveness of different screening strategies.

   (a) No screen.
   (b) Universal biennial screening.
   (c) Personalized strategy 1:

90 ~ 100th percentile	1-yearly	FIT + Stool DNA Test
80 ~ 90th percentile		FIT
60 ~ 80th percentile	2-yearly	
40 ~ 60th percentile	3-yearly	
0 ~ 40th percentile	6-yearly	

   (d) Personalized strategy 2: The same screening modality and inter-screening interval as Strategy C, but 6-yearly for risk group 0 ~ 40th percentile.
   (e) Personalized strategy 3: The sample inter-screening interval as Strategy C, but all had FIT.
   (f) Personalized strategy 4: The sample inter-screening interval as Strategy D, but all had FIT.

11.2.2 Cost-Effectiveness Analysis of Universal and Personalized Colorectal Cancer Screening with FIT

Using the same methodology in cost-effectiveness analysis as mentioned in Chap. 10, the cost-effectiveness analysis of universal FIT screening by different inter-screening intervals, and the personalized screening strategies suggested by personal characteristics (including f-Hb concentration, lifestyle, comorbidity, and genetic and epigenetic factors) was also performed.

11.3 Results

11.3.1 The Multistate And Multifactorial Model

The five-state natural history of colorectal cancer (normal → small adenoma → large adenoma → CRC in the PCDP → CRC in the CP) with state-specific covariates was constructed to build up a risk assessment model on the pathways of adenoma-carcinoma and otherwise de novo (Fig. 11.1b).

Table 11.1 shows the distribution of associated factors and their effects on the transition rates by different transitions. For the incidence of colorectal adenoma, males had a 55% higher risk than females. f-Hb revealed a dose-response relationship with relative risk (RR) from 1.55 for 1–19 ngHb/mL buffer to 10.45 for >450 Hb/mL buffer compared to 1–19 ngHb/mL buffer. Lifestyle (smoking and alcohol drinking), chronic condition (elevated BMI and TG), polygene, and methylation markers (CDH13, CDNK2A, PTGIS, RASSF2, IGTA, RIL, CNRIP1, FBN1, and MAL) also played role for the initiators of adenoma. The RRs of the methylation markers of FBN1, and MAL for the transition from small to large adenoma were 1.68 and 1.20, respectively. Regarding the transition from large adenoma to invasive cancer, P53 mutation carried a 17-fold risk, and the methylation makers of MYOD had an about 14-fold risk. The other three methylation makers (INA, SNCA, SPG20) yielded a 1.75–3.48-fold risk. As far as the transition from the PCDP to the CP is concerned, only the methylation marker of INA was noted (RR = 2.11). The MSH2/MLH1 mutation had a large effect (RR = 55.7) on the de novo pathway, though the mutation was rare (0.0319%).

The estimated clinical weights of the multistep progression to colorectal cancer were expressed by the following five scores

Table 11.1 Relative risk of each factor on different transitions

Characteristics	Classification	% in population		Parameters (Transition rate/RR)	References
Effect on incidence of colorectal adenoma					
Overall transition rate				0.0021	Chen et al. (2003)
Gender	Male	50		1.55	
		F	M		
f-Hb (ng Hb/mL buffer)	Undetected	41.3	40.9	0.72	Yen et al. (2014)
	1–19	33.5	31.6	1.00	
	20–39	13.0	12.9	1.55	
	40–59	4.3	4.8	2.21	
	60–79	2.2	2.4	1.88	
	80–99	1.1	1.4	2.97	
	100–149	1.4	1.5	4.13	
	150–249	1.0	1.4	4.22	
	250–449	0.7	1.0	6.28	
	≥450	1.4	2.2	10.46	
Alcohol drinking	Current or ex-drinker	F: 8.1; M: 45.6		1.18	
		F	M		
BMI (Kg/m²)	≤22	25.9	16.8	1.00	
	22.1–25	33.4	34.4	1.11	
	25.1–27	17.2	23.0	1.27	
	>27	23.6	25.8	1.30	
		F	M		
TG (mg/dL)	≤75	30.9	19.9	1.00	
	75.1–110	25.9	24.0	1.30	
	110.1–165	23.0	25.6	1.35	
	>165	20.2	30.5	1.45	
Smoking	Current and ex-smoker vs. non-smoker	F: 6.9; M: 55.5		1.82	Botteri et al. (2008)
APC mutation		2.5		6.22	Imperiale et al. (2004)
K-ras mutation	Yes vs. No	2.6		2.51	Imperiale et al. (2004)
Polygene	rs6983267	50		Het:1.04, Homo: 1.47	Haiman et al. (2007)
	rs4939827	53		1.15	Broderick et al. (2007)
	rs4779584	19		1.26	Yeager et al. (2008)
	rs16892766	7		1.25	Tomlinson et al. (2008)
	rs10795668	67		1.12	Tomlinson et al. (2008)
	rs3802842	29		1.10	Tenesa et al. (2008)
Methylation markers	CDH13 (H-cadherin)	42.1		1.30	Toyooka et al. (2002)
	CDNK2A(cyclin-dependent kinase inhibitor)	26.7		0.86	Toyota et al. (2000)
	PTGIS (prostanglandin12 synthase)	30.0		1.76	(Frigola et al. 2005)
	RASSF2 (Ras association domain family 2)	42.9		0.96	Akino et al. (2005)
	IGTA (integrin, alpha 4)	75.0		3.83	Ausch et al. (2009)
	RIL (a LIM domain gene mapping to 5q31)	78.6		0.63	Boumber et al. (2007)
	CNRIP1	20.2		1.67	Lind et al. (2011)
	FBN1	13.1		1.69	Lind et al. (2011)
	MAL	7.5		1.84	Lind et al. (2011)
Effect on transition from small-to-large adenoma					

(continued)

Table 11.1 (continued)

Characteristics	Classification	% in population	Parameters (Transition rate/RR)	References
Overall transition			0.13	Chen et al. (2003)
Methylation	FBN1	13.1	1.68	Lind et al. (2011)
	MAL	7.5	1.20	Lind et al. (2011)
Effect on transition from large adenoma to invasive carcinoma				
Overall transition			0.19	Chen et al. (2003)
p53 mutation		1.6	16.95	Imperiale et al. (2004)
Methylation	MYOD (myogenic differentiation 1)	88.2	13.87	Shannon et al. (1999)
	INA	9.7	3.48	Lind et al. (2011)
	SNCA	16.1	1.75	Lind et al. (2011)
	SPG20	14.6	2.19	Lind et al. (2011)
Effect on transition from the PCDP to the CP				
Overall transition			0.30	Chen et al. (2003)
Methylation	INA	9.7	2.11	Lind et al. (2011)
Effect on de novo transition				
Baseline transition			0.00073	Chen et al. (2003)
MSH2/MLH1 mutation		0.0319	55.70	Lin et al. (1998)

$$
\begin{aligned}
\text{Risk score 1} = {} & 0.4383 \times (\text{Male}) - 0.3345 \times (\text{f} - \text{Hb undetected}) + 0.4388 \times (\text{f} - \text{Hb } 20 - 39) + 0.7944 \\
& \times (\text{f} - \text{Hb } 40 - 59) + 0.6308 \times (\text{f} - \text{Hb } 60 - 79) + 1.0894 \times (\text{f} - \text{Hb } 80 - 99) + 1.4185 \\
& \times (\text{f} - \text{Hb } 100 - 149) + 1.4393 \times (\text{f} - \text{Hb } 150 - 249) + 1.8368 \times (\text{f} - \text{Hb } 250 - 449) + 2.3474 \\
& \times (\text{f} - \text{Hb } 450+) + 0.1676 \times (\text{drinking}) + 0.1052 \times (\text{BMI}_{Q2}) + 0.2426 \times (\text{BMI}_{Q3}) + 0.2640 \\
& \times (\text{BMI}_{Q4}) + 0.2594 \times (\text{TG}_{Q2}) + 0.2982 \times (\text{TG}_{Q3}) + 0.3713 \times (\text{TG}_{Q4}) + 0.0392 \\
& \times (\text{Heterozyous rs6983267}) + 0.3853 \times (\text{Homozyous rs6983267}) + 0.599 \\
& \times (\text{Smoking}) + 1.8278 \times (\text{APC}) + 0.9203 \times (k - \text{ras}) + 0.140 \\
& \times (\text{no. of rs4939827 risk alleles}) + 0.231 \times (\text{no. of rs4779584 risk alleles}) + 0.223 \\
& \times (\text{no. of rs168927667 risk alleles}) + 0.113 \times (\text{no. of rs10795668 risk alleles}) + 0.095 \\
& \times (\text{no. of rs3802842 risk alleles}) + 0.261 \times (\text{CDH13}) - 0.149 \times (\text{CDNK2A}) + 0.565 \\
& \times (\text{PTGIS}) - 0.043 \times (\text{RASSF2}) + 1.344 \times (\text{IGTA}) - 0.463 \times (\text{RIL}) + 0.513 \times (\text{CNRIP}) + 0.525 \\
& \times (\text{FBN1}) + 0.610 \times (\text{MAL})
\end{aligned}
$$

$$
\text{Risk score 2} = 0.518 \times (\text{FBN1}) + 0.180 \times (\text{MAL})
$$

$$
\text{Risk score 3} = 2.8303 \times (\text{p53}) + 2.629 \times (\text{MYOD}) + 1.247 \times (\text{INA}) + 0.56 \times (\text{SNCA}) + 0.784 \times (\text{SPG20})
$$

$$
\text{Risk score 4} = 0.747 \times (\text{INA})
$$

$$
\text{Risk score 5} = 4.02 \times (\text{MSH2 / MLH1})
$$

11.3.2 Risk Classification

According to the probability of developing colorectal cancer predicted from the risk scores derived in the previous section, we present the risk score percentile for each specific subject. Figure 11.2 shows the predicted risk of colorectal neoplasm in 20 years for eleven subjects at 95th, 90th, 80th, …, 10th, and fifth risk percentile. At 20-year follow-up, those at 95th percentile were 3.61-fold compared with those at median value. On the opposite, the case at fifth percentile had roughly half of risk compared to the case at median point.

11.3.3 Mean Sojourn Time for Large Adenoma

Our model enables us to predict the mean sojourn time (MST) from large adenoma to invasive carcinoma for subjects with different risk profiles. Table 11.2 shows the estimated mean sojourn time for six cases. The MST varied substantially

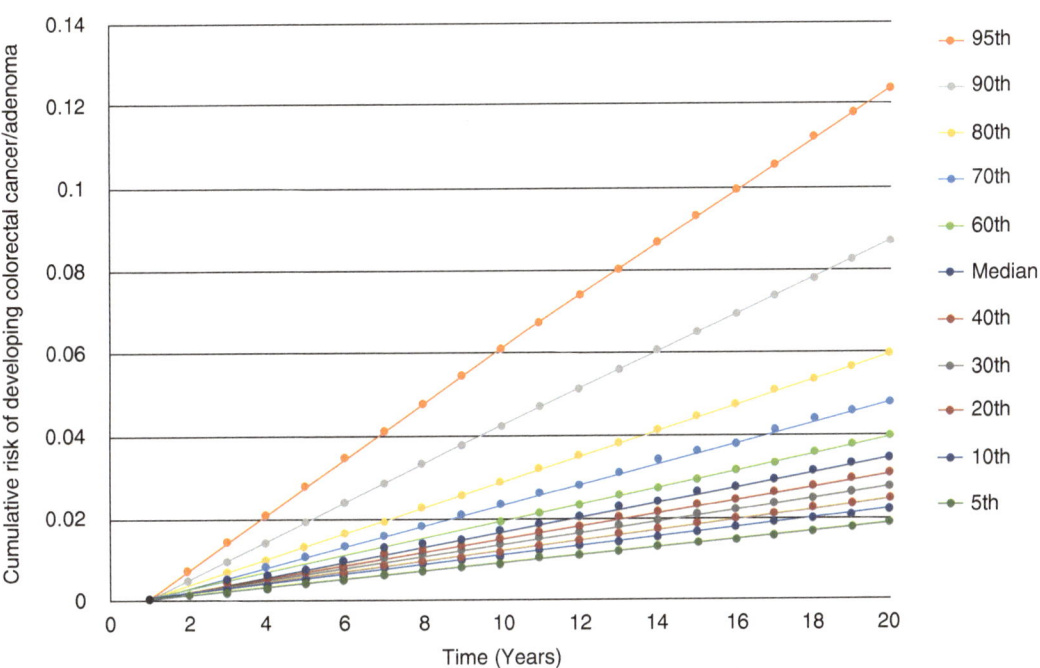

Fig. 11.2 Cumulative risk of developing colorectal neoplasm with 11 cases* in different risk score percentiles. * Risk profiles of subjects

Table 11.2 Mean sojourn times from large adenoma to invasive carcinoma by the combination of different promoters

P53 mutation	Hyper-methylation of myod	Hyper-methylation of INA	Hyper-methylation of SNCA, SPG20	Mean sojourn times (Years)
Yes	Yes	Yes	No	0.15
Yes	Yes	No	No	0.52
Yes	No	No	Yes	1.87
No	Yes	Yes	No	2.52
No	Yes	No	No	8.78
No	No	No	Yes	31.75

for those with different risk profiles. For example, subjects with p53 mutation and hypermethylation of MYOD and INA but not for SNCA and SPG20 had a 0.15-year MST whereas subjects with hypermethylation of MYOD but without INA, SNCA, SPG20, and p53 mutation had about 32-year MST.

11.3.4 Association Between f-Hb Level and Risk Percentile

While f-Hb is an important risk factor as an initiator for the occurrence of colorectal adenoma, the proportion of higher risk percentiles in the cohort increased with an elevated level of f-Hb. Table 11.3 and Fig. 11.2 show the distribution of risk percentiles by level of f-Hb.

11.3.5 Effectiveness of Personalized CRC Screening

Table 11.4 shows the predicted effectiveness of biennial FIT screening and four personalized

strategies in terms of reduction of CRC death compared to no screen. The universal biennial screening was expected to bring down 45% CRC mortality. This figure was close to the personalized screening with varying inter-screening intervals for FIT (Personalized 4: 1-, 2-, and 3-years for the top three 20% bands and 4-years for the bottom 40% risk). However, the latter had lower number of screens for each subject (6.45 ± 3.34) than the biennial program (6.90 ± 0.64). The long interval for the bottom 20% risk group to 6-years (Personalized 3) only resulted in slightly less benefit (RR = 0.56). If stool DNA is provided for the top 10% risk group as a complementary to FIT, the overall mortality reduction was even lower (RR = 0.50 for Personalized 2 and RR = 0.51 for Personalized 1) with an average of 6.45 (±3.34) and 6.05 (±3.65) rounds of screens for Personalized 2 and 1, respectively, for each subject.

As far as the effectiveness on reducing newly diagnosed CRC cases, the reduction of incident CRC for biennial was 37%, which was close to the results of effectiveness with Personalized Strategy 3 and 4 but lower than the two personal-

Table 11.3 The distribution of subjects in different risk percentiles by level of f-Hb

f-Hb (mg Hb/mL buffer)	Risk Percentile N (%)										
	0–9	10–19	20–29	30–39	40–49	50–59	60–69	70–79	80–89	90–100	Total
Undetected	62,588	57,476	53,156	48,667	45,030	41,202	37,317	32,468	25,276	14,051	417,231
	(15.00)	(13.78)	(12.74)	(11.66)	(10.79)	(9.88)	(8.94)	(7.78)	(6.06)	(3.37)	
1–19	30,471	31,796	34,579	35,930	36,259	36,087	35,887	34,606	31,812	20,918	328,345
	(9.28)	(9.68)	(10.53)	(10.94)	(11.04)	(10.99)	(10.93)	(10.54)	(9.69)	(6.37)	
20–39	5571	7469	8322	10,474	12,235	14,081	15,654	17,696	19,810	17,780	129,092
	(4.32)	(5.79)	(6.45)	(8.11)	(9.48)	(10.91)	(12.13)	(13.71)	(15.35)	(13.77)	
40–59	704	1758	1902	2295	3061	4024	5064	6364	8749	10,658	44,579
	(1.58)	(3.94)	(4.27)	(5.15)	(6.87)	(9.03)	(11.36)	(14.28)	(19.63)	(23.91)	
60–79	599	996	1132	1495	1811	2238	2542	3183	3999	4242	22,237
	(2.69)	(4.48)	(5.09)	(6.72)	(8.14)	(10.06)	(11.43)	(14.31)	(17.98)	(19.08)	
80–99	53	285	369	412	555	815	1112	1629	2445	4107	11,782
	(0.45)	(2.42)	(3.13)	(3.50)	(4.71)	(6.92)	(9.44)	(13.83)	(20.75)	(34.86)	
> = 100	14	220	540	727	1049	1553	2424	4054	7909	28,244	46,734
	(0.03)	(0.47)	(1.16)	(1.56)	(2.24)	(3.32)	(5.19)	(8.67)	(16.92)	(60.44)	
Total	100,000	100,000	100,000	100,000	100,000	100,000	100,000	100,000	100,000	100,000	1,000,000

ized strategies 1 and 2, with the orders of reduction being 41% and 40%, respectively.

11.3.6 Cost-Effectiveness Analysis of Universal and Personalized Screening with FIT

The results regarding the cost-effectiveness analysis of personalized screening, universal FIT screening by different inter-screening intervals, and the personalized screening strategies suggested by personal characteristics (including f-Hb concentration, lifestyle, comorbidity, and genetic and epigenetic factors) was provided. The cost-effectiveness of universal FIT screening was cost-saving compared with no screening. Annual FIT (FIT1) and biennial FIT (FIT2) were also cost-saving compared with annual guaiac fecal occult blood test (gFOBT 1). Regarding the prob-

ability of being cost-effective for a series of strategies, both FIT1 and FIT2 had a higher probability (up to 80%) of being cost-effective given the willingness-to-pay (WTP) at $20,000 per life-year gained. Compared with gFOBT1, the probabilities for being cost-effective were estimated at over 80% for both FIT1 and FIT2 at a WTP of $20,000 per life-year gained (LYG).

We found personalized strategies with varying inter-screening interval by FIT but not using DNA markers dominated the biennial screening regime as all the incremental cost-effectiveness ratios (ICERs) were negative. Given WTP at $20,000, personalized strategy with varying inter-screening intervals (1-2-3-4-years) by FIT and for the top 10% subjects combined with DNA testing given the ICER equal to $589 was cost-effective whereas personalized strategy with varying inter-screening intervals (1-2-3-6-years) given the ICER equal to $9308 was not.

Table 11.4 Simulated results for the effectiveness of reducing CRC death with different screening strategies by risk percentile[a]

Risk percent	No screen CRC death	Biennial CRC death	RR	Personalized strategy 1 (FIT and Stool DNA test) CRC death	RR	2 (FIT and Stool DNA test) CRC death	RR	3 (FIT) CRC death	RR	4 (FIT) CRC death	RR
0 ~ 5	523	370	0.7075	376	0.7189	395	0.7553	388	0.7419	389	0.7438
5 ~ 10	600	344	0.5733	374	0.6233	416	0.6933	386	0.6433	380	0.6333
10 ~ 20	1284	764	0.5950	889	0.6924	851	0.6628	900	0.7009	851	0.6628
20 ~ 30	1423	830	0.5833	939	0.6599	894	0.6283	1020	0.7168	895	0.6290
30 ~ 40	1561	892	0.5714	978	0.6265	972	0.6227	1022	0.6547	1030	0.6598
40 ~ 50	1723	985	0.5717	998	0.5792	1047	0.6077	956	0.5548	1002	0.5815
50 ~ 60	1949	1042	0.5346	1186	0.6085	1090	0.5593	1091	0.5598	1111	0.5700
60 ~ 70	2266	1257	0.5547	1208	0.5331	1256	0.5543	1186	0.5234	1185	0.5229
70 ~ 80	2775	1406	0.5067	1503	0.5416	1457	0.5250	1430	0.5153	1408	0.5074
80 ~ 90	3813	1918	0.5030	1873	0.4912	1843	0.4833	1858	0.4873	1841	0.4828
90 ~ 95	2640	1311	0.4966	872	0.3303	880	0.3333	1276	0.4833	1307	0.4951
95 ~ 100	5818	3339	0.5739	2234	0.3840	2199	0.3780	3145	0.5406	3092	0.5315
Overall	26,375	14,458	0.5482	13,430	0.5092	13,300	0.5043	14,658	0.5558	14,491	0.5494
# screens		6.90	0.64	6.05	3.65	6.45	3.34	6.06	3.65	6.45	3.34

[a]Personalized strategy 1: 0 ~ 40th pct.: **6-y**; 40 ~ 60th pct.: 3-y; 60 ~ 80th pct.: 2-y; 80 ~ 100th pct.: 1-y; All with FIT, except FIT combined with Stool DNA test for 90 ~ 100th percentile
Personalized strategy 2: 0 ~ 40th pct.: 4-y; 40 ~ 60th pct.: 3-y; 60 ~ 80th pct.: 2-y; 80 ~ 100th pct.: 1-y; All with FIT, except FIT combined with Stool DNA test for 90 ~ 100th percentile.
Personalized strategy 3: 0 ~ 40th pct.: **6-y**; 40 ~ 60th pct.: 3-y; 60 ~ 80th pct.: 2-y; 80 ~ 100th pct.: 1-y; All with FIT;
Personalized strategy 4: 0 ~ 40th pct.: 4-y; 40 ~ 60th pct.: 3-y; 60 ~ 80th pct.: 2-y; 80 ~ 100th pct.: 1-y; All with FIT.

11.4 Discussion

Individually tailored cancer screening for CRC under the concept of translational research has been proposed to solve many problems of current universal mass screening for CRC. Today, a universal mass screening for CRC has been challenged by lower sensitivity for high-risk group when using FIT and lower specificity for low- or average-risk group when using the costly screening tool such as stool DNA or colonoscopy if one cannot consider the individual risk profile with the incorporation of these new scientific discoveries into a multistep natural course. Therefore, health policy-makers for population-based cancer screening for CRC are often stranded by the modest decline in cancer-specific mortality possibly due to less intensive screening, the late age of early detection, and the neglected use of highly accurate screening technique for high-risk subjects and also puzzled by the alarming increased cost when these new technologies or intensive screening are applied to the low-risk group due to lacking guidance from individual risk profiles.

We provide a solution to such a two-throng problem by demonstrating how to achieve individually tailored cancer screening by making use of the state-of-the-art, using fecal hemoglobin concentration, conventional epidemiological risk factors in combination with genetic research finding with a novel quantitative approach.

Regarding economic consideration, FIT screening strategies compared with no screening were cost-saving. Lengthening the inter-screening interval to 2 years for CRC screening with FIT was cost-saving compared to annual gFOBT and it was also cost-effective when lengthening to 3-year. Personalized screening without considering DNA marker was also cost-saving but personalized screening making allowance for DNA markers may be cost-effective depending on cost of DNA markers and the coverage of risk stratum applied with DNA markers.

In conclusion, our novel method and findings have a perspective and significant implication for personalized medicine on screening, surveillance, and treatment of early colorectal cancer. The proposed concept, methodology, and application have a far-reaching implication for different provinces of scientists, professionals, and health policy-makers involved in the prevention of colorectal cancer. We believe the application of personalized information on f-Hb concentration, genetic markers, and nongenetic factors provides a new avenue for designing individually tailored screening policy for colorectal cancer in the era of big data and precision medicine.

Subject	Risk percentile	Gender	f-Hb (ng Hb/mL buffer)	Alcohol drinking	BMI	TG	Smoking	Mutation				SNP (among6)	Hyper-methylation
								APC	K-ras	p53	MSH2/ MLH1		
1	5th	F	Undetected	N	Q1	Q1	N	N	N	N	N	2	CKNK2, RIL
2	10th	F	1–19	N	Q2	Q4	N	N	N	N	N	4	CDH13, PTGIS, RIL
3	20th	M	1–19	Y	Q2	Q2	N	N	Y	N	N	3	MYOD, RIL
4	30th	F	20–39	N	Q4	Q2	Y	N	N	N	N	6	MYOD, RASSF2, RIL
5	40th	F	1–19	N	Q3	Q2	N	Y	N	N	N	2	CDH13, MYOD, RASSF2, RIL
6	Median	M	60–79	N	Q4	Q3	Y	N	N	N	N	4	CDNK2A, MYOD, RIL, MAL, SPG20
7	60th	F	1–19	N	Q2	Q2	N	N	N	Y	N	4	ITG4, RIL, FBN1, INA, MAL, SPG20
8	70th	M	>450	N	Q1	Q1	N	N	N	N	N	5	CDH13, MYOD, RIL, INA, SNCA, SPG20
9	80th	F	40–60	Y	Q3	Q3	N	N	N	Y	N	3	CDH13, MYOD, RASSF2, ITGA4, RIL, FBN1
10	90th	M	40–60	N	Q3	Q2	N	Y	N	N	N	4	MYOD, RIL, FBN1, SPG20
11	95th	M	1–19	Y	Q3	Q2	Y	N	N	Y	N	5	MYOD, PTGIS, ITGA4, RIL, SNCA, mal

References

Akino K, Toyota M, Suzuki H, et al. The Ras effector RASSF2 is a novel tumor-suppressor gene in human colorectal cancer. Gastroenterology. 2005;129:156–69.

Ausch C, Kim Y-H, Tsuchiya KD, et al. Comparative analysis of PCR-based biomarker assay methods for colorectal polyp detection from fecal DNA. Clin Chem. 2009;55:1559–63.

Bosch LJ, Carvalho B, Fijneman RJ, et al. Molecular tests for colorectal cancer screening. Clin Colorectal Cancer. 2011;10:8–23.

Botteri E, Iodice S, Bagnardi V, et al. Smoking and colorectal cancer: a meta-analysis. JAMA. 2008;300:2765–78.

Boumber YA, Kondo Y, Chen X, et al. RIL, a LIM gene on 5q31, is silenced by methylation in cancer and sensitizes cancer cells to apoptosis. Cancer Res. 2007;67:1997–2005.

Broderick P, Carvajal-Carmona L, Pittman AM, et al. A genome-wide association study shows that common alleles of SMAD7 influence colorectal cancer risk. Nat Genet. 2007;39:1315–7.

Cenin DR, Naber SK, de Weerdt AC, et al. Cost-effectiveness of personalized screening for colorectal Cancer based on polygenic risk and family history. Cancer Epidemiol Prev Biomarkers. 2020;29:10–21.

Chen CD, Yen MF, Wang WM, et al. A case-cohort study for the disease natural history of adenoma-carcinoma and de novo carcinoma and surveillance of colon and rectum after polypectomy: implication for efficacy of colonoscopy. Br J Cancer. 2003;88:1866–73.

Chiu HM, Lee YC, Tu CH, et al. Association between early stage colon neoplasms and false-negative results from the fecal immunochemical test. Clin Gastroenterol Hepatol. 2013;11:832–838.e2.

Cox D, Miller H. The theory of stochastic processes. London: Methuen; 1965.

Frigola J, Munoz M, Clark SJ, et al. Hypermethylation of the prostacyclin synthase (PTGIS) promoter is a frequent event in colorectal cancer and associated with aneuploidy. Oncogene. 2005;24:7320.

Haiman CA, Le Marchand L, Yamamato J, et al. A common genetic risk factor for colorectal and prostate cancer. Nat Genet. 2007;39:954–6.

Imperiale TF, Ransohoff DF, Itzkowitz SH, et al. Fecal DNA versus fecal occult blood for colorectal-cancer screening in an average-risk population. N Engl J Med. 2004;351:2704–14.

Jeon J, Du M, Schoen RE, et al. Determining risk of colorectal cancer and starting age of screening based on lifestyle, environmental, and genetic factors. Gastroenterology. 2018;154:2152–2164.e19.

Lin KM, Shashidharan M, Ternent CA, et al. Colorectal and extracolonic cancer variations in MLH1/MSH2 hereditary nonpolyposis colorectal cancer kindreds and the general population. Dis Colon Rectum. 1998;41:428–33.

Lind GE, Danielsen SA, Ahlquist T, et al. Identification of an epigenetic biomarker panel with high sensitivity and specificity for colorectal cancer and adenomas. Mol Cancer. 2011;10:85.

Shannon B, Kay P, House A, et al. Hypermethylation of the Myf-3 gene in colorectal cancers: associations with pathological features and with microsatellite instability. Int J Cancer. 1999;84:109–13.

Tenesa A, Farrington SM, Prendergast JG, et al. Genome-wide association scan identifies a colorectal cancer susceptibility locus on 11q23 and replicates risk loci at 8q24 and 18q21. Nat Genet. 2008;40:631.

Tomlinson IP, Webb E, Carvajal-Carmona L, et al. A genome-wide association study identifies colorectal cancer susceptibility loci on chromosomes 10p14 and 8q23. 3. Nat Genet. 2008;40:623.

Toyooka S, Toyooka KO, Harada K, et al. Aberrant methylation of the CDH13 (H-cadherin) promoter region in colorectal cancers and adenomas. Cancer Res. 2002;62:3382–6.

Toyota M, Ohe-Toyota M, Ahuja N, et al. Distinct genetic profiles in colorectal tumors with or without the CpG island methylator phenotype. Proc Natl Acad Sci. 2000;97:710–5.

Yeager M, Xiao N, Hayes RB, et al. Comprehensive resequence analysis of a 136 kb region of human chromosome 8q24 associated with prostate and colon cancers. Hum Genet. 2008;124:161–70.

Yen AMF, Chen SLS, Chiu SYH, et al. A new insight into fecal hemoglobin concentration-dependent predictor for colorectal neoplasia. Int J Cancer. 2014;135:1203–12.

Young GP, Bosch LJ. Fecal tests: from blood to molecular markers. Curr Colorectal Cancer Rep. 2011;7:62–70.